Complete PSB!

Study guide and practice test questions for the PSB exam

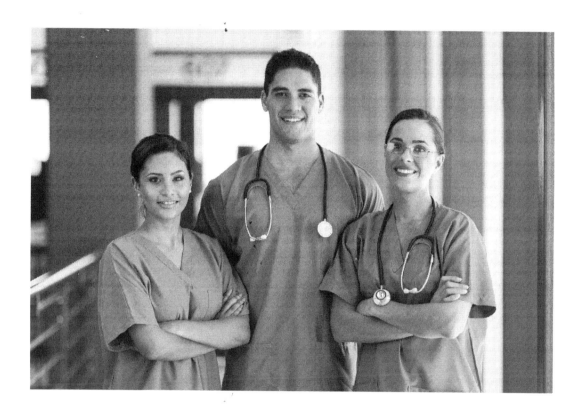

Published by

Blue Butterfly Books™

Copyright Notice

Published by

Blue Butterfly Books™
Victoria BC Canada
Contact us at info@bluebutterflybooks.ca

Printed in the USA

Team Members for this publication

Editor: Sheila Hynes H.BA M.E.S.
Contributor: Dr. C. Gregory
Contributor: Dr. N. Wyatt

Sustainability and Eco-Responsibility

Here at *Blue Butterfly Books*™ , trees are valuable to Mother Earth and the health and wellbeing of everyone. Minimizing our ecological footprint and effect on the environment, we choose Create Space, an eco-responsible printing company.

Electronic routing of our books reduces greenhouse gas emissions, worldwide. When a book order is received, the order is filled at the printing location closest to the client. Using environmentally friendly publishing technology, of the Espresso book printing machine, *Blue Butterfly Books* ™ are printed as they are requested, saving thousands of books, and trees over time. This process offers the stable and viable alternative keeping healthy sustainability of our environment.

All paper is acid-free, and interior paper stock is made from 30% post-consumer waste recycled material. Safe for children, Create Space also verifies the materials used in the print process are all CPSIA-compliant.

By purchasing this *Blue Butterfly Books* ™ , you have supported Full Recovery and Preservation of The Karner Blue Butterfly . Our logo is the Karner Blue Butterfly, Lycaeides melissa samuelis, a rare and beautiful butterfly species whose only flower for propogation is the blue lupin flower. The Karner Butterfly is mostly found in the Great Lakes Region of the U.S.A. Recovery planning is in action, for the return of Karner Blue in Canada led by the National Recovery Strategy. The recovery goals and objectives are aimed at recreating suitable habitats for the butterfly and encourage the growth of blue lupines - the butterfly's natural ideal habitat.

For more info on the Karner Blue Butterfly , feel free to visit:

http://www.albanypinebush.org/conservation/wildlife-management/karner-blue-butterfly-recovery

http://www.wiltonpreserve.org/conservation/karner-blue-butterfly.

http://www.natureconservancy.ca/en/what-we-do/resource-centre/featured-species/karner_blue.html.

Contents

Getting Started

CONGRATULATIONS! By deciding to take the Health Occupations Aptitude Examination (PSB or HOAE) , you have taken the first step toward a great future! Of course, there is no point in taking this important examination unless you intend to do your very best to earn the highest grade you possibly can. That means getting yourself organized and discovering the best approaches, methods and strategies to master the material. Yes, that will require real effort and dedication on your part but if you are willing to focus your energy and devote the study time necessary, before you know it you will be opening that letter of acceptance to the nursing school of your dreams.

We know that taking on a new endeavour can be a little scary, and it is easy to feel unsure of where to begin. That's where we come in. This study guide is designed to help you improve your test-taking skills, show you a few tricks of the trade and increase both your competency and confidence.

Note, however, that the makers of the PSB may have changed the types of questions on the exam as well as exam content after this study guide was created. We recommend that you check with the creators of the test for any new information, and be sure to read the materials supplied on registration carefully.

What is on the PSB

The PSB has these sections: vocabulary, arithmetic, spelling, reading comprehension, form relations and natural sciences. Since how well you score in each of these areas will determine whether or not you get into the best nursing school possible, it is important to be prepared.

Part I - Academic Aptitude

Verbal Sub-test

The Verbal Sub-test contains 30 vocabulary related questions.

Arithmetic Sub-test

The Arithmetic Sub-test contains 30 questions on basic arithmetic.

Nonverbal Sub-test

The Nonverbal Sub-test contains 30 questions that test your comprehension of form relations and ability to manipulate shapes mentally.

Part II – Spelling

This section contains around 30 spelling questions.

Part III - Reading Comprehension

This section contains questions based on a short passage. The questions test comprehension, making inferences and conclusions.

Part IV – Natural Sciences

The section covers introductory level biology, chemistry, and natural science.

How this study guide is organized

This study guide is divided into three sections. The first section, Self-Assessments, which will help you recognize your areas of strength and weaknesses. This will be a boon when it comes to managing your study time most efficiently; there is not much point of focusing on material you already have firmly under control. Instead, taking the self-assessments will show you where that time could be much better spent. In this area you will begin with a few questions to evaluate quickly your understanding of material that is likely to appear on the PSB®. If you do poorly in certain areas, simply work carefully through the tutorials and then try the self-assessment again.

The second section, Tutorials, offers information in each of the content areas, as well as strategies to help you master that material. The tutorials are not intended to be a complete course, but cover general principle. If you find that you do not understand the tutorials, it is recommended that you seek out additional instruction. Note that most Universities recommend students take introductory courses in Math, English and Science before taking the PSB®.

Third, we offer two sets of practice test questions, similar to those on the PSB® V Exam. Again, we cover all modules, so make sure to check with your school!

The PSB® Study Plan

Now that you have made the decision to take the PSB, it is time to get started. Before you do another thing, you will need to figure out a plan of attack. The very best study tip is to start early! The longer the time period you devote to regular study practice, the more likely you will be to retain the material and be able to access it quickly. If you thought that 1x20 is the same as 2x10, guess what? It really is not, when it comes to study time. Reviewing material for just an hour per day over the course of 20 days is far better than studying for two hours a day for only

10 days. The more often you revisit a particular piece of information, the better you will know it. Not only will your grasp and understanding be better, but your ability to reach into your brain and quickly and efficiently pull out the tidbit you need, will be greatly enhanced as well.

The great Chinese scholar and philosopher Confucius believed that true knowledge could be defined as knowing both what you know and what you do not know. The first step in preparing for the PSB® Exam is to assess your strengths and weaknesses. You may already have an idea of what you know and what you do not know, but evaluating yourself using our Self-Assessment modules for each of the three areas, math, english science and reading, will clarify the details.

Making a Study Schedule

To make your study time most productive you will need to develop a study plan. The purpose of the plan is to organize all the bits of pieces of information in such a way that you will not feel overwhelmed. Rome was not built in a day, and learning everything you will need to know to pass the PSB® Exam is going to take time, too. Arranging the material you need to learn into manageable chunks is the best way to go. Each study session should make you feel as though you have succeeded in accomplishing your goal, and your goal is simply to learn what you planned to learn during that particular session. Try to organize the content in such a way that each study session builds on previous ones. That way, you will retain the information, be better able to access it, and review the previous bits and pieces at the same time.

Exam Component	Rate from 1 - 5
Vocabulary	
Arithmetic	
Spelling	
Nonverbal	
Reading Comprehension	
Passage Comprehension	
Drawing inferences & conclusions	

Natural Sciences	
Biology	
Chemistry	
General Science	

Making a Study Schedule

The key to making a study plan is to divide the material you need to learn into manageable size and learn it, while at the same time reviewing the material that you already know.

Using the table above, any scores of three or below, you need to spend time learning, going over and practicing this subject area. A score of four means you need to review the material, but you don't have to spend time re-learning. A score of five and you are OK with just an occasional review before the exam.

A score of zero or one means you really do need to work on this and you should allocate the most time and give it the highest priority. Some students prefer a 5-day plan and others a 10-day plan. It also depends on how much time you have until the exam.

Here is an example of a 5-day plan based on an example from the table above:

Vocabulary: 1   Study 1 hour everyday – review on last day

Arithmetic: 3   Study 1 hour for 2 days then ½ hour a day, then review

Spelling: 4   Review every second day

Biology: 2 Study 1 hour on the first day – then ½ hour everyday

Reading Comprehension: 5   Review for ½ hour every other day

Basic Science: 5   Review for ½ hour every other day

It makes sense to focus your study time on those subjects where you need the most work but unless you create a visual chart for yourself, chances are good you will get confused in no time. First, write out what you need to study and how much time you want to devote to it. Next, consider how many days you have before the test. Plan to take time off from studying on the day before the exam is scheduled. On the last day before the test, you will not learn anything and will probably only confuse yourself. Besides, giving yourself a little break means you will feel fresher on the day of the test.

Make a table that includes slots for the number of days before the test and the number of hours you have available to study each day. We suggest working with half hour and one hour time slots; less than that means you will get set up to study and it will be time to quit, and more than an hour might result in mental fatigue.

Now you are ready to begin filling in the blanks. Give the most time to those subjects you need to study the most. It is also a good idea to assign your weakest subjects the most regular time slots. In fact, even just thirty minutes a day will help lock in the information you need. Of course, those subjects that you know like the back of your hand can be assigned the shortest blocks of time. You will note in the chart we have created that a half hour two or three times a week is all you will need for your strongest subjects.

If you have between two and three hours a day in which to study, you might create a chart that looks something like this to help yourself stay organized:

Day	Subject	Time
Monday		
Study	Vocabulary	1 hour
Study	Biology	1 hour
	½ hour break	
Study	Arithmetic	1 hour
Review	Spelling	½ hour
Tuesday		
Study	Vocabulary	1 hour
Study	Biology	½ hour
	½ hour break	
Study	Arithmetic	½ hour
Review	Spelling	½ hour
Review	Basic Science	½ hour
Wednesday		
Study	Vocabulary	1 hour
Study	Biology	½ hour
	½ hour break	
Study	Arithmetic	½ hour
Review	Basic Science	½ hour
Thursday		
Study	Vocabulary	½ hour
Study	Biology	½ hour
Review	Arithmetic	½ hour
	½ hour break	
Review	Basic Science	½ hour
Review	Spelling	½ hour
Friday		
Review	Vocabulary	½ hour
Review	Biology	½ hour
Review	Arithmetic	½ hour
	½ hour break	
Review	Spelling	½ hour
Review	Biology	½ hour

Tips for making a schedule

Once you set a schedule that works, stick with it! Establish study sessions that are realistic. Blocking out study time that is too long or too short means you will be tempted to cheat. Instead, schedule study sessions that are reasonable and you will set yourself up for success!

Schedule breaks. Breaks are just as important as study time. Work out a rotation of studying and brief breaks that works for you.

Build up study time. If you find it hard to sit still and study for an hour at first, build up to it. Start with 20 minutes, and then take a break. Once you get used to 20-minute study sessions, increase the time to 30 minutes. Gradually work your way up to a full hour.

40 minutes to an hour is optimal. Studying for longer is unlikely to be productive. Studying for periods that are too short won't give you enough time to really learn anything.

Approach math differently. Studying math is different than studying other subjects because you use a different part of your brain. The best way to study math is to practice every day. This will train your mind to think in a mathematical way. If you miss a day or two, the mathematical mind-set is gone and you have to start all over again to build it up.

Vocabulary

BELOW IS A VOCABULARY SELF-ASSESSMENT. The purpose of the self-assessment is to give you a quick baseline score in vocabulary that you can use to make your study schedule as outlined above. It is also extra practice!

The questions below are not the same as you will find on the PSB - that would be too easy! And nobody knows what the questions will be and they change all the time. The questions below cover the same areas as the PSB. So, while the format and exact wording of the questions may differ slightly, and change from year to year, if you can answer the questions below, you will have no problem with the vocabulary section of the PSB.

Since this is a Self-Assessment, and depending on how confident you are with vocabulary, timing is optional. The self-assessment has 15 questions, so allow about 5 minutes to complete this assessment.

The PSB vocabulary is a little different most vocabulary tests. Instead of asking for a definition of a given word, the PSB vocabulary questions give four words and you are asked to choose the word that is most different.

Here is a brief outline of how your score on the self-assessment relates to your understanding of the material.

75% - 100%	Excellent. You have mastered the content
50 – 75%	Good. You have a working knowledge. Even though you can just pass this section, you may want to review the Tutorials and do some extra practice to see if you can improve your mark.
25% - 50%	Below Average. You do not understand the problems. Review the tutorials, and retake this quiz again in a few days, before proceeding to the rest of the practice test questions.
Less than 25%	Poor. You have a very limited understanding. Please review the tutorials, and retake this quiz again in a few days, before proceeding to the rest of the study guide.

After taking the Self-Assessment, use the table above to assess your understanding. If you scored low, read through the tutorials, and make sure you understand everything. Then try again in a few days.

Vocabulary Self-Assessment Answer Sheet

1. A B C D   11. A B C D

2. A B C D   12. A B C D

3. A B C D   13. A B C D

4. A B C D   14. A B C D

5. A B C D   15. A B C D

6. A B C D

7. A B C D

8. A B C D

9. A B C D

10. A B C D

Self-Assessment

Choose the word that is most different in meaning.

1. a. Meager b. Bare c. Scanty d. Obtuse

2. a. Memento b. Gift c. Keepsake d. Memorial

3. a. Necessary b. Optional c. Required d. Essential

4. a. Negotiate b. Bargain c. Haggle d. Scheme

5. a. Expert b. Novice c. Learner d. Beginner

6. a. Narrate b. Relate c. Obfuscate d. Tell

7. a. Negligible b. Overriding c. Unimportant d. Insignificant

8. a. Obstinate b. Adamant c. Ornery d. Stubborn

9. a. Omen b. Premonition c. Unexpected d. Foreboding

10. a. Opulence b. Abundance c. Wealth d. Hoard

11. a. Perplex b. Confuse c. Befuddle d. Astonish

12. a. Parcel b. Bundle c. Luggage d. Package

13. a. Vapid b. Bland c. Insipid d. Tasty

14. a. Plan b. Plight c. Situation d. Scenario

15. a. Feign b. Sham c. Dissemble d. Obviate

Answer Key

1. **D**
2. **B**
3. **B**
4. **D**
5. **A**
6. **C**
7. **B**
8. **C**
9. **C**
10. **D**
11. **D**
12. **C**
13. **D**
14. **A**
15. **D**

How to Improve your Vocabulary

Vocabulary tests can be daunting when you think of the enormous number of words that might come up in the exam. As the exam date draws near, your anxiety will grow because you know that no matter how many words you memorize, chances are, you will still remember so few, and there are so many more to memorize! Here are some tips which you can use to hurdle the big words that may come up in your exam without having to open the dictionary and memorize all the words known to humankind.

Build up and tear apart the big words. Big words, like many other things, are composed of small parts. Some words are made up of many other words. A man who lifts weights for example, is a weight lifter. Words are also made up of word parts called prefixes, suffixes and roots. Often times, we can see the relationship of different words through these parts. A person who is skilled with both hands is ambidextrous. A word with double meaning is ambiguous. A person with two conflicting emotions is ambivalent. Two words with synonymous meanings often have the same root. Bio, a root word derived from Latin is used in words like biography meaning to write about
a person's life, and biology meaning the study of living organisms.

- **Words with double meanings.** Did you know that the word husband not only means a man married to a woman, but also thrift or frugality? Sometimes, words have double meanings. The dictionary meaning, or the denotation of a word is sometimes different from the way we use it or its connotation.

- **Read widely, read deeply and read daily.** The best way to expand your vocabulary is to familiarize yourself with as many words as possible through reading. By reading, you are able to remember words in a proper context and thus, remember its meaning or at the very least, its use. Reading widely would help you get acquainted with words you may never use every day. This is the best strategy without doubt. However, if you are studying for an exam next week, or even tomorrow, it isn't much help! Below you will find a range of different ways to learn new words quickly and efficiently.

- **Remember.** Always remember that big words are easy to understand when divided into smaller parts, and the smaller words will often have several other meanings aside from the one you already know.

- **Be Committed To Learning New Words.** To improve your vocabulary you need to make a commitment to learn new words. Commit to learning at least a word or two a day. You can also get new words by reading books, poems,stories, plays and magazines. Expose yourself to more language to increase the number of new words that you learn.

- **Learn Practical Vocabulary.** As much as possible, learn vocabulary that is associated with what you do and that you can use regularly. For example learn words related to your profession or hobby. Learn as much vocabulary as you can in your favorite subjects.

- **Use New Words Frequently.** When you learn a new word start using it and do so frequently. Repeat it when you are alone and try to use the word as often as you can with people you talk to. You can also use flashcards to practice new words that you learn.

- **Learn the Proper Usage.** If you do not understand the proper usage, look it up and make sure you have it right.

- **Use a Dictionary.** When reading textbooks, novels or assigned readings, keep the dictionary nearby. Also learn how to use online dictionaries and WORD dictionary. When you come across a new word, check for its meaning. If you cannot do so immediately, then you should write it down and check it when possible. This will help you understand what the word means and exactly how best to use it.

- **Learn Word Roots, Prefixes and Suffixes.** English words are usually derived from suffixes, prefixes and roots, which come from Latin, French or Greek. Learning the root or origin of a word helps you easily understand the meaning of the word and other words that are derived from the root. Generally, if you learn the meaning of one root word, you will understand two or three words. This is a great two-for-one strategy. Most prefixes, suffixes, roots and stems are used in two, three or more words, so if you know the root, prefix or suffix, you can guess the meaning of many words.

- **Synonyms and Antonyms.** Most words in the English language have two or three (at least) synonyms and antonyms. For example, "big," in the most common usage, has about seventy-five synonyms and an equal number of antonyms. Understanding the relationships between these words and how they all fit together gives your brain a framework, which makes them easier to learn, remember and recall.

• **Use Flash Cards.** Flash cards are one of the best ways to memorize things. They can be used anywhere and anytime, so you can make use of odd free moments waiting for the bus or waiting in line. Make your own or buy commercially prepared flash cards, and keep them with you all the time.

• **Make Word Lists.** Learning vocabulary, like learning many things, requires repetition. Keep a new words journal in a separate section or separate notebook. Add any words that you look up in the dictionary, as well as from word lists. Review your word lists regularly. Photocopying or printing off word lists from the Internet or handouts is not the same. Actually writing out the word and a few notes on the definition is an important process for imprinting the word in your brain. Writing out the word and definition in your New Word Journal, forces you to concentrate and focus on the new word. Hitting PRINT or pushing he button on the photocopier does not do the same thing.

Nonverbal

BELOW IS A NONVERBAL SKILLS SELF-ASSESSMENT. The purpose of the self-assessment is to give you a quick baseline score in vocabulary that you can use to make your study schedule as outlined above. It is also extra practice!

The questions below are not the same as you will find on the PSB - that would be too easy! And nobody knows what the questions will be and they change all the time. The questions below cover the same areas as the PSB however. So, while the format and exact wording of the questions may differ slightly, and change from year to year, if you can answer the questions below, you will have no problem with the nonverbal section of the PSB.

Since this is a Self-Assessment, and depending on how confident you are with Nonverbal questions, timing is optional. The PSB has 30 questions, to be answered in 30 minutes. The self-assessment has 10 questions, so allow about 10 minutes to complete this assessment.

The self-assessment is designed to give you a baseline score in the different areas covered. Here is a brief outline of how your score on the self-assessment relates to your understanding of the material.

Here is a brief outline of how your score on the self-assessment relates to your understanding of the material.

80% - 100%	Excellent. You have mastered the content
60 – 79%	Good. You have a working knowledge. Even though you can just pass this section, you may want to review the Tutorials and do some extra practice to see if you can improve your mark.
40% - 59%	Below Average. You do not understand the problems. Review the tutorials, and retake this quiz again in a few days, before proceeding to the rest of the practice test questions.

Less than 40%	Poor. You have a very limited understanding of non-verbal problems. Please review the Tutorials, and retake this quiz again in a few days, before proceeding to the rest of the study guide.

After taking the Self-Assessment, use the table above to assess your understanding. If you scored low, read through the tutorials, and make sure you understand everything. Then try again in a few days.

Nonverbal Answer Sheet

1. (A) (B) (C) (D)

2. (A) (B) (C) (D)

3. (A) (B) (C) (D)

4. (A) (B) (C) (D)

5. (A) (B) (C) (D)

6. (A) (B) (C) (D)

7. (A) (B) (C) (D)

8. (A) (B) (C) (D)

9. (A) (B) (C) (D)

10. (A) (B) (C) (D)

Self-Assessment

Select the figure with the same relationship.

1.

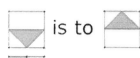 is to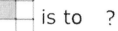

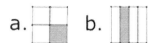 is to ?

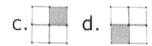

2.

☐ is to ⌐⌐

⬠ is to ?

3.

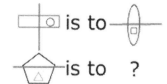 is to ?

4.

⬜ is to ⬜

◇ is to ?

a. 🌐 b. ⬛

c. ⬡ d. ⬜

5.

▯ is to ▭

◯ is to ?

a. ◯ b. ▷

c. ◉ d. ◯▷

6.

▯ is to ◯

⬡ is to ?

a. △ b. ◻

c. △ d. ▯

7. Which does not belong?

a. Slant

b. Lean

c. Tilt

d. Incline

8. Which of the following does not belong?

a. CD

b. OP

c. LM

d. BD

9. Which of the following does not belong?

a. 121212

b. 141414

c. 151415

d. 292929

10. Complete the sequence.

Big Bigger Biggest :: Small Smaller ____

a. Tiny

b. Large

c. Medium

d. Smallest

Answer Key

1. D
The relationship is the same figure flipped vertically, so the best choice is D.

2. C
The relation is the same figure with the bottom half removed.

3. D
The first pair is a rectangle with a circle inside and then an oval with a square inside. The given figures in the second pair has a triangle inside, so the match will be the circle with a square inside.

4. B
The relation is two upright figures in the first set, and 2 horizontal figures in the second set.

5. C
The first pair contains a box with a circle inside, and the same figure on its side.

6. C
The inside and larger shapes are reversed.

7. B
This is a word meaning relationship. Lean is not a synonym for any of the choices.

8. D
BD is not a sequence of consecutive letters.

9. C
This is a repetition pattern. All of the choices repeat a 2-letter sequence except C.

10. D
All the words are comparative adjectives.

Spelling

THIS SECTION CONTAINS A SPELLING SELF-ASSESSMENT. The questions in the self-assessment are not the same as you will find on the PSB - that would be too easy! And nobody knows what the questions will be and they change all the time. Mostly, the changes consist of substituting new questions for old, but the changes also can be new question formats or styles, changes to the number of questions in each section, changes to the time limits for each section, and combining sections. So, while the format and exact wording of the questions may differ slightly, and changes from year to year, if you can answer the questions below, you will have no problem with the spelling section of the PSB.

Spelling Self-Assessment

The purpose of the self-assessment is:

- Identify your strengths and weaknesses.

- Develop your personalized study plan (see Chapter 1)

- Get accustomed to the PSB format

- Extra practice – the self-assessments are almost a full 3rd practice test!

- Provide a baseline score for preparing your study schedule.

Since this is a Self-assessment, and depending on how confident you are with Spelling, timing yourself is optional. The PSB has 30 questions, to be answered in 40 minutes. This self-assessment has 15 questions, so allow 15 minutes to complete.

Once complete, use the table below to assess your understanding of the content, and prepare your study schedule described in chapter 1. If you scored low, read through the tutorials, and make sure you understand everything. Then try again in a few days.

80% - 100%	Excellent. You have mastered the content
60 – 79%	Good. You have a working knowledge. Even though you can just pass this section, you may want to review the Tutorials and do some extra practice to see if you can improve your mark.
40% - 59%	Below Average. You do not understand the content. Review the tutorials, and retake this quiz again in a few days, before proceeding to the rest of the practice test questions.
Less than 40%	Poor. You have a very limited understanding. Please review the Tutorials, and retake this quiz again in a few days, before proceeding to the rest of the study guide.

Spelling Self-Assessment Answer Sheet

1. (A) (B) (C) (D)   11. (A) (B) (C) (D)

2. (A) (B) (C) (D)   12. (A) (B) (C) (D)

3. (A) (B) (C) (D)   13. (A) (B) (C) (D)

4. (A) (B) (C) (D)   14. (A) (B) (C) (D)

5. (A) (B) (C) (D)   15. (A) (B) (C) (D)

6. (A) (B) (C) (D)

7. (A) (B) (C) (D)

8. (A) (B) (C) (D)

9. (A) (B) (C) (D)

10. (A) (B) (C) (D)

Self-Assessment

1. Choose the correct spelling.

    a. Weather

    b. Weathur

    c. Wether

    d. None of the above

2. Choose the correct spelling.

    a. Withdrawl

    b. Withdrawal

    c. Withdrawel

    d. Witdrawal

3. Choose the correct spelling.

    a. Yatch

    b. Yache

    c. Yaute

    d. Yacht

4. Choose the correct spelling.

    a. Yeild

    b. Yielde

    c. Yield

    d. Yeelde

5. Choose the correct spelling.

    a. Warrant

    b. Warrent

    c. Warent

    d. Warant

6. Choose the correct spelling.

    a. Thorou

    b. Thurough

    c. Thorough

    d. Thorogh

7. Choose the correct spelling.

    a. Tomorow

    b. Tomorrow

    c. Tommorow

    d. Tommorrow

8. Choose the correct spelling.

    a. Unicke

    b. Uniqe

    c. Unique

    d. None of the Above.

9. Choose the correct spelling.

    a. Unice

    b. Usable

    c. Ussable

    d. Usabble

10. Choose the correct spelling.

    a. Usually

    b. Usualy

    c. Ususally

    d. Ussually

11. Choose the correct spelling.

    a. Vacoom

    b. Vaccoum

    c. Vacuum

    d. Vacum

12. Choose the correct spelling.

    a. Vengance

    b. Vengeance

    c. Vengeace

    d. Vengece

13. Choose the correct spelling.

    a. Villain

    b. Vilain

    c. Villan

    d. Vilin

14. Choose the correct spelling.

    a. Vollume

    b. Volume

    c. Volum

    d. None of the Above.

15. Choose the correct spelling.

    a. Cemettary

    b. Cemetary

    c. Cemettery

    d. Cemetery

Answer Key

1. A
2. B
3. D
4. C
5. A
6. C
7. B
8. C
9. B
10. A
11. C
12. B
13. A
14. B
15. D

Reading Comprehension

THIS SECTION CONTAINS A READING SELF-ASSESSMENT AND TUTORIALS. The Tutorials are designed to familiarize general principles and the self-assessment contains general questions similar to the reading questions likely to be on the PSB exam, but are not intended to be identical to the exam questions. Many Universities recommend that students take an introductory courses before taking the PSB Exam. The tutorials are not designed to be a complete reading course, and it is assumed that students have some familiarity with reading comprehension questions. If you do not understand parts of the tutorial, or find the tutorial difficult, it is recommended that you seek out additional instruction.

Tour of the PSB Reading Content

Below is a detailed list of the types of reading questions likely to appear on the PSB.

- Drawing logical conclusions

- Identify the author's intent to persuade, inform, entertain, or otherwise

- Make predictions

- Analyze and evaluate the use of text structure to solve problems or identify sequences

- Identify the characteristics of a passage types (narrative, expository, technical, persuasive).

- Follow directions

- Give the definition of a word from context

- Find specific information from a different types of communication (memo, posted notice etc.)

- Find given information from a table of contents or index

- Find information from a graphic (chart or similar, graphic representation)

- Identify and use scale, legends on a sample map

The questions below are not the same as you will find on the PSB - that would be too easy! And nobody knows what the questions will be and they change all the time. Mostly the changes consist of substituting new questions for old, but the changes can be new question formats or styles, changes to the number of questions in each section, changes to the time limits for each section and combining sections. Below are general reading questions that cover the same areas as the PSB. So, while the format and exact wording of the questions may differ slightly, and change from year to year, if you can answer the questions below, you will have no problem with the reading section of the PSB.

Reading Self-Assessment

The purpose of the self-assessment is:

- Identify your strengths and weaknesses.

- Develop your personalized study plan (above)

- Get accustomed to the PSB format

- Extra practice – the self-assessments are almost a full 3rd practice test!

- Provide a baseline score for preparing your study schedule.

Since this is a Self-assessment, and depending on how confident you are with Reading Comprehension, timing is optional. The self-assessment has 12 questions, so allow about 15 minutes to complete this assessment.

Once complete, use the table below to assess your understanding of the content, and prepare your study schedule described in chapter 1.

80% - 100%	Excellent. You have mastered the content
60 – 79%	Good. You have a working knowledge. Even though you can just pass this section, you may want to review the Tutorials and do some extra practice to see if you can improve your mark.

40% - 59%	Below Average. You do not understand the problems. Review the tutorials, and retake this quiz again in a few days, before proceeding to the rest of the practice test questions.
Less than 40%	Poor. You have a very limited understanding of the reading comprehension problems. Please review the Tutorials, and retake this quiz again in a few days, before proceeding to the rest of the study guide.

After taking the Self-Assessment, use the table above to assess your understanding. If you scored low, read through the tutorials, and make sure you understand everything. Then try again in a few days.

Reading Comprehension Self-Assessment Answer Sheet

1. (A) (B) (C) (D)   11. (A) (B) (C) (D)

2. (A) (B) (C) (D)   12. (A) (B) (C) (D)

3. (A) (B) (C) (D)   13. (A) (B) (C) (D)

4. (A) (B) (C) (D)   14. (A) (B) (C) (D)

5. (A) (B) (C) (D)   15. (A) (B) (C) (D)

6. (A) (B) (C) (D)   16. (A) (B) (C) (D)

7. (A) (B) (C) (D)   17. (A) (B) (C) (D)

8. (A) (B) (C) (D)   18. (A) (B) (C) (D)

9. (A) (B) (C) (D)   19. (A) (B) (C) (D)

10. (A) (B) (C) (D)   20. (A) (B) (C) (D)

Self-Assessment

Questions 1 – 4 refer to the following passage.

Passage 1 - The Immune System

An immune system is a system of biological structures and processes that protects against disease by identifying and killing pathogens and other threats. The immune system can detect a wide variety of agents, from viruses to parasitic worms, and distinguish them from the organism's own healthy cells and tissues. Detection is complicated as pathogens evolve rapidly to avoid the immune system defences, and successfully infect their hosts.

The human immune system consists of many types of proteins, cells, organs, and tissues, which interact in an elaborate and dynamic network. As part of this more complex immune response, the human immune system adapts over time to recognize specific pathogens more efficiently. This adaptation process is called "adaptive immunity" or "acquired immunity" and creates immunological memory. Immunological memory created from a primary response to a specific pathogen, provides an enhanced response to future encounters with that same pathogen. This process of acquired immunity is the basis of vaccination. [1]

1. What can we infer from the first paragraph in this passage?

a. When a person's body fights off the flu, this is the immune system in action

b. When a person's immune system functions correctly, they avoid all sicknesses and injuries

c. When a person's immune system is weak, a person will likely get a terminal disease

d. When a person's body fights off a cold, this is the circulatory system in action

2. The immune system's primary function is to:

a. Strengthen the bones

b. Protect against disease

c. Improve respiration

d. Improve circulation

3. Based on the passage, what can we say about evolution's role in the immune system?

a. Evolution of the immune system is an important factor in the immune system's efficiency

b. Evolution causes a person to die, thus killing the pathogen

c. Evolution plays no known role in immunity

d. The least evolved earth species have better immunity

4. Which sentence below, taken from the passage, tell us the main idea of the passage?

a. The human immune system consists of many types of proteins, cells, organs, and tissues, which interact in an elaborate and dynamic network.

b. An immune system is a system of biological structures and processes that protects against disease by identifying and killing pathogens and other threats.

c. The immune system can detect a wide variety of agents, from viruses to parasitic worms, and distinguish them from the organism's own healthy cells and tissues.

d. None of these express the main idea.

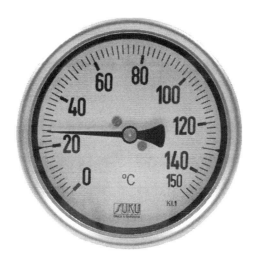

5. Consider the gauge above. What is the temperature?

a. 26⁰ C

b. 23⁰ C

c. 22⁰ C

d. 25⁰ C

Questions 6 – 9 refer to the following passage.

Passage 2 - White Blood Cells

White blood cells (WBCs), or leukocytes (also spelled "leucocytes"), are cells of the immune system that defend the body against both infectious disease and foreign material. Five different and diverse types of leukocytes exist, but they are all produced and derived from a powerful cell in the bone marrow known as a hematopoietic stem cell. Leukocytes are found throughout the body, including the blood and lymphatic system.

The number of WBCs in the blood is often an indicator of disease. There are normally between 4×10^9 and 1.1×10^{10} white blood cells in a liter of blood, making up about 1% of blood in a healthy adult. The physical properties of white blood cells, such as volume, conductivity, and granularity, changes due to the presence of immature cells, or malignant cells.

The name white blood cell derives from the fact that after processing a blood sample in a centrifuge, the white cells are typically a thin, white layer of nucleated cells. The scientific term leukocyte directly reflects this description, derived from Greek leukos (white), and kytos (cell). [2]

6. What can we infer from the first paragraph in this selection?

   a. Red blood cells are not as important as white blood cells

   b. White blood cells are the culprits in most infectious diseases

   c. White blood cells are essential to fight off infectious diseases

   d. Red blood cells are essential to fight off infectious diseases

7. What can we say about the number of white blood cells in a liter of blood?

   a. They make up about 1% of a healthy adult's blood

   b. There are 10^{10} WBCs in a healthy adult's blood

   c. The number varies according to age

   d. They are a thin white layer of nucleated cells

8. What is a more scientific term for "white blood cell"?

a. Red blood cell

b. Anthrocyte

c. Leukocyte

d. Leukemia

9. Can the number of leukocytes indicate cancer?

a. Yes, the white blood cell count can indicate disease.

b. No, the white blood cell count is not a reliable indicator.

c. Disease may indicate a high white blood cell count.

d. None of the choices are correct.

Questions 10 - 12 refer to the following passage.

Passage 3 - Thunderstorms I

Warm air is less dense than cool air, so warm air rises within cooler air like a hot air balloon or warm water in an ocean current. Clouds form as warm air carrying moisture rises. As the warm air rises, it cools, and the moist water vapor begins to condense. This releases energy that keeps the air warmer than its surroundings, and as a result, continues to rise. If enough instability is present in the atmosphere, this process will continue long enough for cumulonimbus clouds to form, which support lightning and thunder. All thunderstorms, regardless of type, go through three stages: the cumulus stage, the mature stage, and the dissipation stage. Depending on the conditions in the atmosphere, these three stages can take anywhere from 20 minutes to several hours. [3]

10. This passage tells us

a. Warm air is denser than cool air

b. All thunderstorms go through three stages

c. Thunderstorms may occur without clouds present

d. The stages of a thunderstorm conclude within just a few minutes

11. When warm air rises through colder air, it results in

    a. Evaporation

    b. Humidity

    c. Clear skies

    d. Condensation

12. This passage is an example of what type of writing?

    a. Narrative

    b. Expository

    c. Persuasive

    d. Technical Manual

The Civil War

The Civil War began on April 12, 1861. The first shots of the Civil War were fired in Fort Sumter, South Carolina. Note that even though more American lives were lost in the Civil War than in any other war, not one person died on that first day. The war began because eleven Southern states seceded from the Union and tried to start their own government, The Confederate States of America.

Why did the states secede? The issue of slavery was a primary cause of the Civil War. The eleven southern states relied heavily on their slaves to foster their farming and plantation lifestyles. The northern states, many of whom had already abolished slavery, did not feel that the southern states should have slaves. The north wanted to free all the slaves and President Lincoln's goal was to both end slavery and preserve the Union. He had Congress declare war on the Confederacy on April 14, 1862. For four long, blood soaked years, the North and South fought.

From 1861 to mid 1863, it seemed as if the South would win this war. However, on July 1, 1863, an epic three day battle was waged on a field in Gettysburg, Pennsylvania. Gettysburg is remembered for being the bloodiest battle in American history. At the end of the three days, the North turned the tide of the war in their favor. The North then went on to dominate the South for the remainder of the war. Most well remembered might be General Sherman's "March to The Sea," where he famously led the Union Army through Georgia and the Carolinas, burning and destroying everything in their path.

In 1865, the Union army invaded and captured the Confederate capital of Richmond Virginia. Robert E. Lee, leader of the Confederacy surrendered to General Ulysses S. Grant, leader of the Union forces, on April 9, 1865. The Civil War was over and the Union was preserved.

13. What does secede mean?

    a. To break away from
    b. To accomplish
    c. To join
    d. To lose

14. Which of the following statements summarizes a FACT from the passage?

    a. Congress declared war and then the Battle of Fort Sumter began.
    b. Congress declared war after shots were fired at Fort Sumter.
    c. President Lincoln was pro slavery
    d. President Lincoln was at Fort Sumter with Congress

15. Which event finally led the Confederacy to surrender?

    a. The battle of Gettysburg
    b. The battle of Bull Run
    c. The invasion of the confederate capital of Richmond
    d. Sherman's March to the Sea

16. The word abolish as used in this passage most nearly means?

    a. To ban
    b. To polish
    c. To support
    d. To destroy

Scottish Wind Farms

The Scottish Government has a targeted plan of generating 100% of Scotland's electricity through renewable energy by 2020. Renewable energy sources include sun, water and wind power. Scotland uses all forms but its fastest growing energy is wind energy. Wind power is generated through the use of wind turbines, placed onshore and offshore. Wind turbines that are grouped together in large numbers are called wind farms. A majority of Scottish citizens say that the wind farms are necessary to meet current and future energy needs, and would like to see an increase in the number of wind farms. They cite the fact that wind energy does not cause pollution, there are low operational costs, and most importantly due to the definition of renewable energy it cannot be depleted.

17. What is Scotland's fastest growing source of renewable energy?

    a. Solar Panels

    b. Hydroelectric

    c. Wind

    d. Fossil Fuels

18. Why do the majority of Scottish citizens agree with the Government's plan?

    a. Their concern for current and future energy needs

    b. Because of the low operational costs

    c. Because they are out of sight

    d. Because it provides jobs

Scottish Wind Farms II

However, there is still a public debate concerning the use of wind farms to generate energy. The most cited argument against wind energy is that the upfront investment is expensive. They also argue that it is aesthetically displeasing, they are noisy, and they create a serious threat to wildlife in the area. While wind energy is renewable, or cannot be depleted, it does not mean that wind is always available. Wind is fluctuating, or intermittent, and therefore not suited to meet the base amount of energy demand, meaning if there is no wind then no energy is being created.

19. What is the biggest argument against wind energy?

    a. The turbines are noisy

    b. The turbines endanger wildlife

    c. The turbines are expensive to build

    d. They are aesthetically displeasing

20. What is the best way to describe this article's description of wind energy?

      a. Loud and ever present

      b. The cheapest form of renewable energy

      c. The only source of renewable energy in Scotland

      d. Clean and renewable but fluctuating

Answer Key

1. A
The passage does not mention the flu specifically, however we know the flu is a pathogen (A bacterium, virus, or other microorganism that can cause disease). Therefore, we can infer, when a person's body fights off the flu, this is the immune system in action.

2. B
The immune system's primary function is to protect against disease.

3. A
The passage refers to evolution of the immune system being important for efficiency. In paragraph three, there is a discussion of adaptive and acquired immunity, where the immune system "remembers" pathogens.
We can conclude, evolution of the immune system is an important factor in the immune system's efficiency.

4. B
The sentence that expresses the main idea of the passage is, "An immune system is a system of biological structures and processes that protects against disease by identifying and killing pathogens and other threats."

5. A
The temperature gauge is showing 26^{0}

6. C
We can infer white blood cells are essential to fight off infectious diseases, from the passage, "cells of the immune system that defend the body against both infectious disease and foreign material."

7. A
We can say the number of white blood cells in a liter of blood make up about 1% of a healthy adult's blood. This is a fact-based question that is easy and fast to answer. The question asks about a percentage. You can quickly and easily scan the passage for the percent sign, or the word percent and find the answer.

8. C
A more scientific term for "white blood cell" is leukocyte, from the first paragraph, first sentence of the passage.

9. A
The white blood cell count can indicate disease (cancer). We know this from the last sentence of paragraph two, "The physical properties of white blood cells, such

as volume, conductivity, and granularity, changes due to the presence of immature cells, or malignant cells."

10. B

All thunderstorms will go through three stages. This is taken directly from the text, "All thunderstorms, regardless of type, go through three stages: the cumulus stage, the mature stage, and the dissipation stage."

11. D

Condensation. From the passage, "As the warm air rises, it cools, and the moist water vapor begins to condense."

12. B

This passage is an example of a expository writing, which is intended to explain or describe something.

13. A

Secede most nearly means to break away from because the 11 states wanted to leave the United States and form their own country.

Option B is incorrect because the states were not accomplishing anything. Option C is incorrect because the states were trying to leave the USA not join it. Option D is incorrect because the states seceded before they lost the war.

14. B

Look at the dates in the passage. The shots were fired on April 12 and Congress declared war on April 14.

Option C is incorrect because the passage states that Lincoln was against slavery. Option D is incorrect because it never mentions who was or was not at Fort Sumter.

15. C

The passage states that Lee surrendered to Grant after the capture of the capital of the Confederacy, which is Richmond.

Option A is incorrect because the war continued for 2 years after Gettysburg. Option B is incorrect because that battle is not mentioned in the passage. Option D is incorrect because the capture of the capital occurred after the march to the sea.

16. A

When the passage said that the North had *abolished* slavery, it implies that slaves were no longer allowed in the North. In essence slavery was banned.

Option B makes no sense relative to the context of the passage. Option C is incorrect because we know the North was fighting slavery, not for it. Option D is incorrect because slavery is not a tangible thing that can be destroyed. It is a practice that had to be outlawed or banned.

17. C
Wind is the highest source of renewable energy in Scotland. The other choices are either not mentioned at all or not mentioned in the context for how fast they are growing.

18. A
Most Scottish citizens agree with the Government's plan due to the concern for current and future needs.

Choice B is a good choice but not why the majority agree. Choice C is meant to mislead the as they are clearly in sight. Choice D is a good 'common sense' choice but mentioned specifically in the text.

19. C
The up-front cost is expensive.
The other choices may appear to be correct, and even be common sense, but they are not specifically mentioned in the paragraph.

20. D
The best way to describe the paragraphs description of wind energy is clean and renewable but fluctuating.
The other choices are good descriptions of wind energy, but not the best way to describe the article.

Help with Reading Comprehension

At first sight, reading comprehension tests look challenging especially if you are given long essays to answer only two to three questions. While reading, you might notice your attention wandering, or you may feel sleepy. Do not be discouraged because there are various tactics and long range strategies that make comprehending even long, boring essays easier.

Your friends before your foes. It is always best to tackle essays or passages with familiar subjects rather than those with unfamiliar ones. This approach applies the same logic as tackling easy questions before hard ones. Skip passages that do not interest you and leave them for later when there is more time left.

Don't use 'special' reading techniques. This is not the time for speed-reading or anything like that – just plain ordinary reading – not too slow and not too fast.

Read through the entire passage and the questions before you do anything. Many students try reading the questions first and then looking for answers in the passage thinking this approach is more efficient. What these students do not realize is that it is often hard to navigate in unfamiliar roads. If you do not familiarize yourself with the passage first, looking for answers become not only time-consuming but also dangerous because you might miss the context of the answer you are looking for. If you read the questions first you will only confuse yourself and lose valuable time.

Familiarize yourself with reading comprehension questions. If you are familiar with the common types of reading comprehension questions, you are able to take note of important parts of the passage, saving time. There are six major kinds of reading comprehension questions.

- **Main Idea**- Questions that ask for the central thought or significance of the passage.

- **Specific Details** - Questions that asks for explicitly stated ideas.

- **Drawing Inferences** - Questions that ask for a statement's intended meaning.

- **Tone or Attitude** - Questions that test your ability to sense the emotional state of the author.

- **Context Meaning** – Questions that ask for the meaning of a word depending on the context.

- **Technique** – Questions that ask for the method of organization or the writing style of the author.

Read. Read. Read. The best preparation for reading comprehension tests is always to read, read and read. If you are not used to reading lengthy passages, you will probably lose concentration. Increase your attention span by making a habit out of reading.

Reading Comprehension tests become less daunting when you have trained yourself to read and understand fast. Always remember that it is easier to understand passages you are interested in. Do not read through passages hastily. Make mental notes of ideas that you think might be asked.

Reading Comprehension Strategy

When facing the reading comprehension section of a standardized test, you need a strategy to be successful. You want to keep several steps in mind:

- **First, make a note of the time and the number of sections.** Time your work accordingly. Typically, four to five minutes per section is sufficient. Second, read the directions for each selection thoroughly before beginning (and listen well to any additional verbal instructions, as they will often clarify obscure or confusing written guidelines). You must know exactly how to do what you're about to do!

- **Now you're ready to begin reading the selection.** Read the passage carefully, noting significant characters or events on a scratch sheet of paper or underlining on the test sheet. Many students find making a basic list in the margins helpful. Quickly jot down or underline one-word summaries of characters, notable happenings, numbers, or key ideas. This will help you better retain information and focus wandering thoughts. Remember, however, that your main goal in doing this is to find the information that answers the questions. Even if you find the passage interesting, remember your goal and work fast but stay on track.

- **Now read the question and all the choices.** Now you have read the passage, have a general idea of the main ideas, and have marked the important points. Read the question and all the choices. Never choose an answer without reading them all! Questions are often designed to confuse – stay focussed and clear. Usually the answer choices will focus on one or two facts or inferences from the passage. Keep these clear in your mind.

- **Search for the answer.** With a very general idea of what the different choices are, go back to the passage and scan for the relevant information. Watch for big words, unusual or unique words. These make your job easier as you can scan the text for the particular word.

- **Mark the Answer.** Now you have the key information the question is looking for. Go back to the question, quickly scan the choices and mark the correct one.

Understand and practice the different types of standardized reading comprehension tests. See the list above for the different types. Typically, there will be several questions dealing with facts from the selection, a couple more inference questions dealing with logical consequences of those facts, and periodically an application-oriented question surfaces to force you to make connections with what you already know. Some students prefer to answer the questions as listed, and feel classifying the question and then ordering is wasting precious time. Other students prefer to answer the different types of questions in order of how easy or difficult they are. The choice is yours and do whatever works for you. If you want to try answering in order of difficulty, here is a recommended order, answer fact questions first; they're easily found within the passage. Tackle inference problems next, after re-reading the question(s) as many times as you need to. Application or 'best guess' questions usually take the longest, so save them for last.

Use the practice tests to try out both ways of answering and see what works for you.

For more help with reading comprehension, see Multiple Choice Secrets at www.multiple-choice.ca

Mathematics

THIS SECTION CONTAINS A MATH SELF-ASSESSMENT AND TUTORIALS. The Tutorials are designed to familiarize general principles and the Self-Assessment contains general questions similar to the math questions likely to be on the PSB exam, but are not intended to be identical to the exam questions. Many Universities recommend that students take an introductory Math course before taking the PSB Exam. The tutorials are not designed to be a complete math course, and it is assumed that students have some familiarity with math. If you do not understand parts of the tutorial, or find the tutorial difficult, it is recommended that you seek out additional instruction.

Tour of the PSB Mathematics Content

The PSB Mathematics section has 30 questions. Below is a detailed list of the mathematics topics likely to appear on the PSB. Make sure that you understand these topics at the very minimum.

- Convert decimals, percent, roman numerals and fractions

- Solve word problems

- Calculate percent and ratio

- Operations using fractions, percent and fractions

- Determine quantities and/or total cost from information given

- Analyze and interpret tables, graphs and charts

- Convert and estimate metric measurements

- Understand and solve simple algebra problems

The questions in the self-assessment are not the same as you will find on the PSB - that would be too easy! And nobody knows what the questions will be and they change all the time. Mostly, the changes consist of substituting new questions for old, but the changes also can be new question formats or styles, changes to the number of questions in each section, changes to the time limits for each section, and combining sections. So, while the format and exact wording of the questions may differ slightly, and changes from year to year, if you can answer the questions below, you will have no problem with the Math section of the PSB.

Mathematics Self-Assessment

The purpose of the self-assessment is:

- Identify your strengths and weaknesses.

- Develop your personalized study plan (above)

- Get accustomed to the PSB format

- Extra practice – the self-assessments are almost a full 3rd practice test!

- Provide a baseline score for preparing your study schedule.

Since this is a Self-assessment, and depending on how confident you are with Math, timing yourself is optional. The PSB has 30 questions, to be answered in 30 minutes. This self-assessment has 30 questions, so allow 30 minutes to complete.

Once complete, use the table below to assess your understanding of the content, and prepare your study schedule described in chapter 1.

80% - 100%	Excellent. You have mastered the content
60 – 79%	Good. You have a working knowledge. Even though you can just pass this section, you may want to review the Tutorials and do some extra practice to see if you can improve your mark.

40% - 59%	Below Average. You do not understand the problems. Review the tutorials, and retake this quiz again in a few days, before proceeding to the rest of the practice test questions.
Less than 40%	Poor. You have a very limited understanding of the problems. Please review the Tutorials, and retake this quiz again in a few days, before proceeding to the rest of the study guide.

Math Self-Assessment Answer Sheet

1. (A) (B) (C) (D)   11. (A) (B) (C) (D)   21. (A) (B) (C) (D)

2. (A) (B) (C) (D)   12. (A) (B) (C) (D)   22. (A) (B) (C) (D)

3. (A) (B) (C) (D)   13. (A) (B) (C) (D)   23. (A) (B) (C) (D)

4. (A) (B) (C) (D)   14. (A) (B) (C) (D)   24. (A) (B) (C) (D)

5. (A) (B) (C) (D)   15. (A) (B) (C) (D)   25. (A) (B) (C) (D)

6. (A) (B) (C) (D)   16. (A) (B) (C) (D)   26. (A) (B) (C) (D)

7. (A) (B) (C) (D)   17. (A) (B) (C) (D)   27. (A) (B) (C) (D)

8. (A) (B) (C) (D)   18. (A) (B) (C) (D)   28. (A) (B) (C) (D)

9. (A) (B) (C) (D)   19. (A) (B) (C) (D)   29. (A) (B) (C) (D)

10. (A) (B) (C) (D)   20. (A) (B) (C) (D)   30. (A) (B) (C) (D)

Self-Assessment

1. Translate the following into an equation: six times a number plus five.

    a. 6X + 5

    b. 6(X+5)

    c. 5X + 6

    d. (6 * 5) + 5

2. Brad has agreed to buy everyone a Coke. Each drink costs $1.89, and there are 5 friends. Estimate Brad's cost.

    a. $7

    b. $8

    c. $10

    d. $12

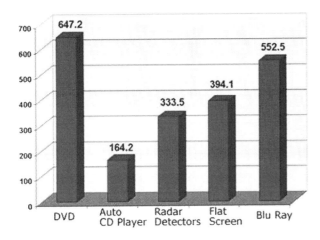

3. Consider the graph above.
What is the third best-selling product?

    a. Radar Detectors

    b. Flat Screen

    c. Blu Ray

    d. Auto CD Players

4. Which two products are the closest in the number of sales?

    a. Blu Ray and Flat Screen TV

    b. Flat Screen TV and Radar Detectors

    c. Radar Detectors and Auto CD Players

    d. DVD players and Blu Ray

5. Sarah weighs 25 pounds more than Tony. If together they weigh 205 pounds, how much will Sarah weigh approximately in kilograms? Assume 1 pound = 0.4535 kilograms.

    a. 41

    b. 48

    c. 50

    d. 52

6. A building is 15 m long and 20 m wide and 10 m high. What is the volume of the building?

    a. 45 m^3

    b. $3,000 \text{ m}^3$

    c. 1500 m^3

    d. 300 m^3

7. 15 is what percent of 200?

    a. 7.5%

    b. 15%

    c. 20%

    d. 17.50%

8. A boy has 5 red balls, 3 white balls and 2 yellow balls. What percent of the balls are yellow?

    a. 2%

    b. 8%

    c. 20%

    d. 12%

9. Add 10% of 300 to 50% of 20

    a. 50

    b. 40

    c. 60

    d. 45

10. Convert 75% to a fraction.

    a. 2/100

    b. 85/100

    c. 3/4

    d. 4/7

11. Multiply 3 by 25% of 40

    a. 75

    b. 30

    c. 68

    d. 35

12. What is 10% of 30 multiplied by 75% of 200?

    a. 450

    b. 750

    c. 20

    d. 45

13. Convert 4/20 to percent

    a. 25%

    b. 20%

    c. 40%

    d. 30%

14. Convert 0.55 to percent

    a. 45%

    b. 15%

    c. 75%

    d. 55%

15. A man buys an item for $420 and has a balance of $3000.00. How much did he have before?

    a. $2,580

    b. $3,420

    c. $2,420

    d. $342

16. What is the best approximate solution for 1.135 - 113.5?

    a. -110

    b. 100

    c. -90

    d. 110

17. Solve 3/4 + 2/4 + 1.2

    a. 1 1/7

    b. 2 3/4

    c. 2 9/20

    d. 3 1/4

18. The physician orders 40 mg Depo-Medrol; 80 mg/ml is on hand. How many milliliters will you give?

    a. 0.5 ml

    b. 0.80 ml

    c. 0.25 ml

    d. 0.40 ml

19. The physician orders 750 mg Tagamet liquid; 1500 mg/tsp is on hand. How many teaspoons will you give?

    a. 0.75 tsp

    b. 0.5 tsp

    c. 1 tsp

    d. 0.55 tsp

20. Convert 10 kg. to grams.

    a. 10,000 grams

    b. 1,000 grams

    c. 100 grams

    d. 10.11 grams

21. 1 gallon = _____ liter(s).

    a. 1 liter

    b. 3.785 liters

    c. 37.85 liters

    d. 4.5 liters

22. Convert 2.5 liters to milliliters.

    a. 1,050 ml.

    b. 2,500 ml.

    c. 2,050 ml.

    d. 1,500 ml.

23. Convert 210 mg. to grams.

    a. 0.21 mg.

    b. 2.1 g.

    c. 0.21 g.

    d. 2.12 g.

24. Convert 10 pounds to kilograms.

    a. 4.54 kg.

    b. 11.25 kg.

    c. 15 kg.

    d. 10.25 kg.

25. Convert 0.539 grams to milligrams.

    a. 539 g.

    b. 539 mg.

    c. 53.9 mg.

    d. 0.53 g.

26. The average weight of 13 students in a class of 15 (two were absent that day) is 42 kg. When the remaining two are weighed, the average became 42.7 kg. If one of the remaining students weighs 48 kg., how much does the other weigh?

    a. 44.7 kg.

    b. 45.6 kg.

    c. 46.5 kg.

    d. 47.4 kg.

27. The total expense of building a fence around a square-shaped field is $2000 at a rate of $5 per meter. What is the length of one side?

    a. 40 meters

    b. 80 meters

    c. 100 meters

    d. 320 meters

28. There were some oranges in a basket. By adding 8/5 of the total to the basket, the new total is 130. How many oranges were in the basket?

    a. 60

    b. 50

    c. 40

    d. 35

29. 3 boys are asked to clean a surface that is 4 ft2. If the surface is divided equally among the boys, what size will each cl**ean?**

      a. 1 ft 6 inches^2

      b. 14 inches^2

      c. 1 ft 2 inches^2

      d. 1 ft^2 48 inches^2

30. A person earns \$25,000 per month and pays \$9,000 income tax per year. The Government increased income tax by 0.5% per month and his monthly earning was increased \$11,000. How much more income tax will he pay per month?

      a. \$1260

      b. \$1050

      c. \$750

      d. \$510

Answer Key

1. B

Six times a number plus five is the same as saying six times (a number plus five). Or, 6 * (a number plus five). Let X be the number so, 6(X+5).

2. C

If there are 5 friends and each drink costs $1.89, we can round up to $2 per drink and estimate the total cost at, 5 X $2 = $10.
The actual, cost is 5 X $1.89 = $9.45.

3. B

Flat Screen TVs are the third best-selling product.

4. B

The two products that are closest in the number of sales, are Flat Screen TVs and Radar Detectors.

5. D

Let us denote Sarah's weight by "x". Then, since she weighs 25 pounds more than Tony, Tony will be x-25. They together weigh 205 pounds which means that the sum of the two representations will be equal to 205:

Sarah : x

Tony : x - 25

x + (x - 25) = 205 ... by arranging this equation we have:

x + x - 25 = 205

2x - 25 = 205 ... we add 25 to each side in order to have x term alone:

2x - 25 + 25 = 205 + 25

2x = 230

x = 230/2

x = 115 pounds so Sarah weighs 115 pounds. Since 1 pound is 0.4535 kilograms, we need to multiply 115 by 0.4535 in order to have her weight in kilograms:

x = 115 • 0.4535 = 52.1525 kilograms - this is equal to 52 when rounded to the nearest whole number.

6. B
Formula for volume of a shape is L x W x H = 15 x 20 x 10 = 3,000 m³

7. A
15/200 = X/100
200X = (15 * 100)
1500/20 Cancel zeroes in the numerator and denominator
15/2 = 7.5%.

Notice that the questions asks, What 15 is what percent of 200?   The question does not ask, what is 15% of 200! The answers are very different.

8. C
Total no. of balls = 10, no. of yellow balls = 2, so = 2/10 X 100 = 20%

9. B
10% of 300 = 30 and 50% of 20 = 10 so 30 + 1- = 40.

10. C
75%= 75/100 = 3/4
11. B
25% of 40 = 10 and 10 x 3 = 30

12. A
10% of 30 = 3 and 75% of 200 = 150, 3 X 150 = 450
13. B
4/20 X 100 = 1/5 X 100 = 20%

14. D
0.55 X 100 = 55%

15. B
(Amount Spent) $420 + $3000 (Balance) = $3420

16. A
1.135 -113.5 = -113.5 + 1-135 = -112.37. Best approximate = -110

17. C
3/4 + 2/4 + 1.2, first convert the decimal to fraction, = 3/4 + 2/4 + 1 1/5 = ¾ + 2/4 + 6/5 = (find common denominator) (15 + 10 + 24)/20 = 49/20 = 2 9/20

18. A
Set up the formula -
Dose ordered/Dose on hand X Quantity/1 = Dosage

40 mg/80 mg X 1 ML/1 = 40/80 = 0.5 mL

19. B
Set up the formula -
Dose ordered/Dose on hand X Quantity/1 = Dosage
750 mg/1500 mg X 1 tsp/1 = 750/1500 = 0.5 tsp

20. A
1kg = 1,000 g and 10 kg = 10 x 1,000 = 10,000 g

21. B
1 US gallon = 3.78541178 liters

22. B
1 liter = 1,000 milliliters, 2.5 liters = 2.5 x 1,000 = 2,500 milliliters

23. C
1,000 mg = 1 g, 210 mg = 210/1000 = 0.21 g.   Be careful of Choice A, (0.21 mg.)
The numbers are the same but the units are different.

24. A
1 pound = 0.45 kg, 10 pounds = 4.53592, or about 4.54 kg.   When multiplying a
decimal by 10, move the decimal point one place to the left.

25. B 1 g = 1,000 mg. 0.539 g = 0.539 x 1000 = 539 mg.

26. C
Total weight of 13 students with average 42 will be = 42•13 = 546 kg.

The total weight of the remaining 2 will be found by subtracting the total weight
of 13 students from the total weight of 15 students: 640.5 - 546 = 94.5 kg.

94.5 = the total weight of two students. One of these students weigh 48 kg, so;

The weight of the other will be = 94.5 – 48 = 46.5 kg

27. C
Total expense is $2000 and we are informed that $5 is spent per meter.
Combining these two information, we know that the total length of the fence is
2000/5 = 400 meters.

The fence is built around a square shaped field. If one side of the square is "a,"
the perimeter of the square is "4a." Here, the perimeter is equal to 400 meters.
So,

$400 = 4a$

$100 = a$ - this means that one side of the square is equal to 100 meters

28. B
Let the number of oranges in the basket before additions = x

Then: $X + 8x/5 = 130$

$5x + 8x = 650$

$650 = 13x$

$X = 50$

29. D
1 foot is equal to 12 inches. So 1 ft^2 = 12•12 in^2

4 ft^2 = 4•12•12 in^2 = 576 in^2

This amount of surface area is divided equally among 3 boys.

Each boy will clean 576/3 = 192 in^2

192 in^2 = 144 in^2 + 48 in^2; 144 in^2 = 1 ft^2

So, each boy will clean 1 ft^2 and 48 in^2

30. D
The income tax per year is $9,000. So, the income tax per month is 9,000/12 = $750.

This person earns $25,000 per month and pays $750 income tax. We need to find the rate of the income tax:

Tax rate: 750•100/25,000 = 3%

Government increased this rate by 0.5% so it became 3.5%.

The income of the person per month is increased $11,000 so it became: $25,000 + $11,000 = $36,000.

The new monthly income tax is: 36,000•3.5/100 = $1260.

Amount of increase in tax per month is: $1260 - $750 = $510.

Metric Conversion – A Quick Tutorial

Conversion between metric and standard units can be tricky since the units of distance, volume, area and temperature can seem rather arbitrary when compared to one another. Although the metric system (using SI units) is the standard system of measure in most parts of the world many countries still use at least some of their traditional units of measure. In North America those units come from the old British system.

When measuring distance the relation between metric and standard units looks like this:

0.039 in	1 millimeter	1 inch	25.4 mm
3.28 ft	1 meter	1 foot	.305 m
0.621 mi	1 kilometer	1 mile	1.61 km

Here, you can see that 1 millimeter is equal to .039 inches and 1 inch equals 25.4 millimeters.

When measuring **area** the relation between metric and standard looks like this:

.0016 in^2	1 square millimeter	1 square inch	645.2 mm^2
10.764 ft^2	1 square meter	1 square foot	.093 m^2
.386 mi^2	1 square kilometer	1 square mile	2.59 km^2
2.47 ac	hectare	1 acre	.405 ha

Similarly, when measuring **volume** the relation between metric and standard units looks like this:

3034 fl oz	1 milliliter	1 fluid ounce	29.57 ml
.0264 gal	1 liter	1 gallon	3.785 L
35.314 ft^3	1 cubic meter	1 cubic foot	.028 m^3

When measuring **weight** and **mass** the relation between metric and standard units looks like this:

.035 oz	1 gram	1 ounce	28.35 g
2.202 lbs	1 kilogram	1 pound	.454 kg
1.103 T	1 metric ton	1 ton	.907 t

Note that in science, the metric units of grams and kilograms are always used to denote the mass of an object rather than its weight.

In predominantly metric countries the standard unit of temperature is degrees

Celsius while in countries with only limited use of the metric system, such as the United States, degrees Fahrenheit is used. This chart shows the difference between Fahrenheit and Celsius:

0° Celsius	32° Fahrenheit
10° Celsius	50° Fahrenheit
20° Celsius	68° Fahrenheit
30° Celsius	86° Fahrenheit
40° Celsius	104° Fahrenheit
50° Celsius	122° Fahrenheit
60° Celsius	140° Fahrenheit
70° Celsius	158° Fahrenheit
80° Celsius	176° Fahrenheit
90° Celsius	194° Fahrenheit
100° Celsius	212° Fahrenheit

As you can see 0° C is freezing while 32° F is freezing. Similarity 100° C is boiling while the Fahrenheit system takes until 212° F. To convert from Celsius to Fahrenheit you need to multiply the temperature in Celsius by 1.8 and then add 32 to it. (x° F = (y° C*1.8) + 32) To convert from Fahrenheit to Celsius you do the opposite. First subtract 32 from the temperature then divide by 1.8. (x° C = (y° -32) / 1.8)

Fraction Tips, Tricks and Shortcuts

When you are writing an exam, time is precious, and anything you can do to answer questions faster, is a real advantage. Here are some ideas, shortcuts, tips and tricks that can speed up answering fraction problems.

Remember that a fraction is just a number which names a portion of something. For instance, instead of having a whole pie, a fraction says you have a part of a pie--such as a half of one or a fourth of one.

Two digits make up a fraction. The digit on top is known as the numerator. The digit on the bottom is known as the denominator. To remember which is which, just remember that "denominator" and "down" both start with a "d." And the "downstairs" number is the denominator. So for instance, in ½, the numerator is the 1 and the denominator (or "downstairs") number is the 2.

- It's easy to add two fractions if they have the same denominator. Just add the digits on top and leave the bottom one the same: 1/10 + 6/10 = 7/10.

- It's the same with subtracting fractions with the same denominator: 7/10 - 6/10 = 1/10.

☐ Adding and subtracting fractions with different denominators is a little more complicated. First, you have to get the problem so that they do have the same denominators. One of the easiest ways to do this is to multiply the denominators: For 2/5 + 1/2 multiply 5 by 2. Now you have a denominator of 10. But now you have to change the top numbers too. Since you multiplied the 5 in 2/5 by 2, you also multiply the 2 by 2, to get 4. So the first number is now 4/10. Since you multiplied the second number times 5, you also multiply its top number by 5, to get a final fraction of 5/10. Now you can add 5 and 4 together to get a final sum of 9/10.

☐ Sometimes you'll be asked to reduce a fraction to its simplest form. This means getting it to where the only common factor of the numerator and denominator is 1. Think of it this way: Numerators and denominators are brothers that must be treated the same. If you do something to one, you must do it to the other, or it's just not fair. For instance, if you divide your numerator by 2, then you should also divide the denominator by the same. Let's take an example: The fraction 2/10 . This is not reduced to its simplest terms because there is a number that will divide evenly into both: the number 2. We want to make it so that the only number that will divide evenly into both is 1. What can we divide into 2 to get 1? The number 2, of course! Now to be "fair," we have to do the same thing to the denominator: Divide 2 into 10 and you get 5. So our new, reduced fraction is 1/5.

☐ In some ways, multiplying fractions is the easiest of all: Just multiply the two top numbers and then multiply the two bottom numbers. For instance, with this problem:
2/5 X 2/3 you multiply 2 by 2 and get a top number of 4; then multiply 5 by 3 and get a bottom number of 15. Your answer is 4/15.

☐ Dividing fractions is a bit more involved, but still not too hard. You once again multiply, but only AFTER you have turned the second fraction upside-down. To divide ⅞ by ½, turn the ½ into 2/1, then multiply the top numbers and multiply the bottom numbers: ⅞ X 2/1 gives us 14 on top and 8 on the bottom.

Converting Fractions to Decimals

There are a couple of ways to become good at converting fractions to decimals. One -- the one that will make you the fastest in basic math skills -- is to learn some basic fraction facts. It's a good idea, if you're good at memory, to memorize the following:

1/100 is "one hundredth," expressed as a decimal, it's .01.

1/50 is "two hundredths," expressed as a decimal, it's .02.

1/25 is "one twenty-fifths" or "four hundredths," expressed as a decimal, it's .04.

1/20 is "one twentieth" or ""five hundredths," expressed as a decimal, it's .05.

1/10 is "one tenth," expressed as a decimal, it's .1.

1/8 is "one eighth," or "one hundred twenty-five thousandths," expressed as a decimal, it's .125.

1/5 is "one fifth," or "two tenths," expressed as a decimal, it's .2.

1/4 is "one fourth" or "twenty-five hundredths," expressed as a decimal, it's .25.

1/3 is "one third" or "thirty-three hundredths," expressed as a decimal, it's .33.

1/2 is "one half" or "five tenths," expressed as a decimal, it's .5.

3/4 is "three fourths," or "seventy-five hundredths," expressed as a decimal, it's .75.

Of course, if you're no good at memorization, another good technique for converting a fraction to a decimal is to manipulate it so that the fraction's denominator is 10, 10, 1000, or some other power of 10. Here's an example: We'll start with ¾. What is the first number in the 4 "times table" that you can multiply and get a multiple of 10? Can you multiply 4 by something to get 10? No. Can you multiply it by something to get 100? Yes! 4 X 25 is 100. So let's take that 25 and multiply it by the numerator in our fraction ¾. The numerator is 3, and 3 X 25 is 75. We'll move the decimal in 75 all the way to the left, and we find that ¾ is .75.

We'll do another one: 1/5. Again, we want to find a power of 10 that 5 goes into evenly. Will 5 go into 10? Yes! It goes 2 times. So we'll take that 2 and multiply it by our numerator, 1, and we get 2. We move the decimal in 2 all the way to the left and find that 1/5 is equal to .2.

Converting Fractions to Percent

Working with either fractions or percents can be intimidating enough. But converting from one to the other? That's a genuine nightmare for those who are not math wizards. However, it doesn't have to be that way. Here are two ways to make it easier and faster to convert a fraction to a percent.

  ☐   First, you might remember that a fraction is nothing more than a division problem: you're dividing the bottom number into the top number. So for instance, if we start with a fraction 1/10, we are making a division problem with the 10 on the outside the bracket and the 1 on the inside. As you remember from your lessons on dividing by decimals, since 10 won't go into 1, you add a decimal and make it 10 into 1.0. 10 into 10 goes 1 time, and since it's behind the decimal, it's .1. And how do we say .1? We say "one tenth," which is exactly what we started with: 1/10. So we have a number we can work with now: .1. When we're dealing with percents, though, we're dealing strictly with hundredths (not tenths). You remember from studying decimals that adding a zero to the right of the number on the right side of the decimal does not change the value. Therefore, we can change .1 into .10 and have the same number--except now it's expressed as hundredths. We have 10 hundredths. That's ten out of 100--which is just another way of saying ten percent (ten per hundred or ten out of 100). In other words .1 = .10 = 10 percent. Remember, if you're changing from a decimal to a percent, get rid of the decimal on the left and replace it with a percent mark on the right: 10%. Let's review those steps again: Divide 10 into 1. Since 10 doesn't go into 1, turn 1 into 1.0. Now divide 10 into 1.0. Since 10 goes into 10 1 time, put it there and add your decimal to make it .1. Since a percent is always "hundredths," let's change .1 into .10. Then remove the decimal on the left and replace with a percent sign on the right. The answer is 10%.

☐ If you're doing these conversions on a multiple-choice test, here's an idea that might be even easier and faster. Let's say you have a fraction of 1/8 and you're asked what the percent is. Since we know that "percent" means hundredths, ask yourself what number we can multiply 8 by to get 100. Since there is no number, ask what number gets us close to 100. That number is 12: 8 X 12 = 96. So it gets us a little less than 100. Now, whatever you do to the denominator, you have to do to the numerator. Let's multiply 1 X 12 and we get 12. However, since 96 is a little less than 100, we know that our answer will be a percent a little MORE than 12%. So if your possible answers on the multiple-choice test are these:

a) 8.5%   b) 19%   c) 12.5%   d) 25%

then we know the answer is c) 12.5%, because it's a little MORE than the 12 we got in our math problem above.

Another way to look at this, using multiple choice strategy is you know the answer will be "about" 12. Looking at the other choices, they are all either too large or too small and can be eliminated right away.

This was an easy example to demonstrate, so don't be fooled! You probably won't get such an easy question on your exam, but the principle holds just the same. By estimating your answer quickly, you can eliminate choices immediately and save precious exam time.

Decimal Tips, Tricks and Shortcuts

Converting Decimals to Fractions

One of the most important tricks for correctly converting a decimal to a fraction doesn't involve math at all. It's simply to learn to say the decimal correctly. If you say "point one" or "point 25" for .1 and .25, you'll have more trouble getting the conversion correct. But if you know that it's called "one tenth" and "twenty-five hundredths," you're on the way to a correct conversion. That's because, if you know your fractions, you know that "one tenth" looks like this: 1/10. And "twenty-five hundredths" looks like this: 25/100.

Even if you have digits before the decimal, such as 3.4, learning how to say the word will help you with the conversion into a fraction. It's not "three point four," it's "three and four tenths." Knowing this, you know that the fraction which looks like "three and four tenths" is 3 4/10.

Of course, your conversion is not complete until you reduce the fraction to its lowest terms: It's not 25/100, but 1/4.

Converting Decimals to Percent

Changing a decimal to a percent is easy if you remember one math formula: multiply by 100. For instance, if you start with .45, you change it to a percent by simply multiplying it by 100. You then wind up with 45. Add the % sign to the end and you get 45%.

That seems easy enough, right? Here think of it this way: You just take out the decimal and stick in a percent sign on the opposite sign. In other words, the decimal on the left is replaced by the % on the right.

It doesn't work quite that easily if the decimal is in the middle of the number. Let's use 3.7 as an example. Here, take out the decimal in the middle and replace it with a 0 % at the end. So 3.7 converted to decimal is 370%.

Percent Tips, Tricks and Shortcuts

Percent problems are not nearly as scary as they appear, if you remember this neat trick:

Draw a cross as in:

Portion	Percent
Whole	100

In the upper left, write PORTION. In the bottom left write WHOLE. In the top right, write PERCENT and in the bottom right, write 100. Whatever your problem is, you will leave blank the unknown, and fill in the other four parts. For example, let's suppose your problem is: Find 10% of 50. Since we know the 10% part, we put 10 in the percent corner. Since the whole number in our problem is 50, we put that in the corner marked whole. You always put 100 underneath the percent, so we leave it as is, which leaves only the top left corner blank. This is where we'll put our answer. Now simply multiply the two corner numbers that are NOT 100. Here, it's 10 X 50. That gives us 500. Now multiply this by the remaining corner, or 100, to get a final answer of 5. 5 is the number that goes in the upper-left corner, and is your final solution.

Another hint to remember: Percents are the same thing as hundredths in decimals. So .45 is the same as 45 hundredths or 45 percent.

Converting Percents to Decimals

Percents are simply a specific type of decimals, so it should be no surprise that converting between the two is actually fairly simple. Here are a few tricks and shortcuts to keep in mind:

- Remember that percent literally means "per 100" or "for every 100." So when you speak of 30% you're saying 30 for every 100 or the fraction 30/100. In basic math, you learned that fractions that have 10 or 100 as the denominator can easily be turned into a decimal. 30/100 is thirty hundredths, or expressed as a decimal, .30.
- Another way to look at it: To convert a percent to a decimal, simply divide the number by 100. So for instance, if the percent is 47%, divide 47 by 100. The result will be .47. Get rid of the % mark and you're done.
- Remember that the easiest way of dividing by 100 is by moving your decimal two spots to the left.

Converting Percents to Fractions

Converting percents to fractions is easy. After all, a percent is nothing except a type of fraction; it tells you what part of 100 that you're talking about. Here are some simple ideas for making the conversion from a percent to a fraction:

- ☐ If the percent is a whole number -- say 34% -- then simply write a fraction with 100 as the denominator (the bottom number). Then put the percentage itself on top. So 34% becomes 34/100.
- ☐ Now reduce as you would reduce any percent. In this case, by dividing 2 into 34 and 2 into 100, you get 17/50.
- ☐ If your percent is not a whole number -- say 3.4% --then convert it to a decimal expressed as hundredths. 3.4 is the same as 3.40 (or 3 and forty hundredths). Now ask yourself how you would express "three and forty hundredths" as a fraction. It would, of course, be 3 40/100. Reduce this and it becomes 3 2/5.

How to Answer Basic Math Multiple Choice

Math is the one section where you need to make sure that you understand the processes before you ever tackle it. That's because the time allowed on the math portion is typically so short that there's not much room for error. You have to be fast and accurate. It's imperative that before the test day arrives, you've learned all of the main formulas that will be used, and then to create your own problems (and solve them).

On the actual test day, use the "Plug-Check-Check" strategy. Here's how it goes.

Read the problem, but not the answers. You'll want to work the problem first and come up with your own answers. If you did the work right, you should find your answer among the choices given.

If you need help with the problem, plug actual numbers into the variables given. You'll find it easier to work with numbers than it is to work with letters. For instance, if the question asks, "If Y-4 is 2 more than Z, then Y+5 is how much more than Z?" try selecting a value for Y. Let's take 6. Your question now becomes, "If 6-4 is 2 more than Z, then 6 plus 5 is how much more than Z?" Now your answer should be easier to work with.

Check the answer choices to see if your answer matches one of those. If so, select it.

If no answer matches the one you got, re-check your math, but this time, use a different method. In math, it's common for there to be more than one way to solve a problem. As a simple example, if you multiplied 12 X 13 and did not get an answer that matches one of the answer choices, you might try adding 13 together 12 different times and see if you get a good answer.

Math Multiple Choice Strategy

The two strategies for working with basic math multiple choice are Estimation and Elimination.

Math Strategy 1 - Estimation.

Just like it sounds, try to estimate an approximate answer first. Then look at the choices.

Math Strategy 2 - Elimination.

For every question, no matter what type, eliminating obviously incorrect answers narrows the possible choices. Elimination is probably the most powerful strategy for answering multiple choice.

Here are a few basic math examples of how this works.

Solve 2/3 + 5/12

    a. 9/17
    b. 3/11
    c. 7/12
    d. 1 1/12

First estimate the answer. 2/3 is more than half and 5/12 is about half, so the answer is going to be very close to 1.

Next, Eliminate. Choice A is about 1/2 and can be eliminated, Choice B is very small, less than 1/2 and can be eliminated. Choice C is close to 1/2 and can be eliminated. Leaving only Choice D, which is just over 1.

Work through the solution, a common denominator is needed, a number which both 3 and 12 will divide into.
2/3 = 8/12. So, 8 + 5/12 = 13/12 = 1 1/12

Choice D is correct.

Solve 4/5 – 2/3

  a. 2/2

  b. 2/13

  c. 1

  d. 2/15

You can eliminate Choice A, because it is 1 and since both of the numbers are close to one, the difference is going to be very small. You can eliminate Choice C for the same reason.

Next, look at the denominators. Since 5 and 3 don't go in to 13, you can eliminate Choice B as well.

That leaves Choice D.

Checking the answer, the common denominator will be 15.   So 12-10/15 = 2/15. Choice D is correct.

Fractions shortcut - Cancelling out

In any operation with fractions, if the numerator of one fractions has a common multiple with the denominator of the other, you can cancel out. This saves time and simplifies the problem quickly, making it easier to manage.

Solve 2/15 ÷ 4/5

  a. 6/65

  b. 6/75

  c. 5/12

  d. 1/6

To divide fractions, we multiply the first fraction with the inverse of the second fraction. Therefore we have 2/15 x 5/4. The numerator of the first fraction, 2, shares a multiple with the denominator of the second fraction, 4, which is 2.

These cancel out, which gives, 1/3 x 1/2 = 1/6. Cancelling Out solved the questions very quickly, but we can still use multiple choice strategies to answer. Choice B can be eliminated because 75 is too large a denominator. Choice C can be eliminated because 5 and 15 don't go into 12.

Choice D is correct.

Decimal Multiple Choice strategy and Shortcuts

Multiplying decimals gives a very quick way to estimate and eliminate choices. Anytime that you multiply decimals, it is going to give a answer with the same number of decimal places as the combined operands.

So for example,

2.38 X 1.2 will produce a number with three places of decimal, which is 2.856. Here are a few examples with step-by-step explanation:

Solve 2.06 x 1.2

    a. 24.82

    b. 2.482

    c. 24.72

    d. 2.472

This is a simple question, but even before you start calculating, you can eliminate several choices. When multiplying decimals, there will always be as many numbers behind the decimal place in the answer as the sum of the ones in the initial problem, so Choice A and C can be eliminated.

The correct answer is D: 2.06 x 1.2 = 2.472

Solve 20.0 ÷ 2.5

    a. 12.05

    b. 9.25

    c. 8.3

    d. 8

First estimate the answer to be around 10, and eliminate Choice A. And since it'd also be an even number, you can eliminate Choice B and C., leaving only choice D.

The correct Answer is D: 20.0 ÷ 2.5 = 8

How to Solve Word Problems

Most students find math word problems difficult. Tackling word problems is much easier if you have a systematic approach which we outline below.

Here is the biggest tip for studying word problems.

Practice regularly and systematically. Sounds simple and easy right? Yes it is, and yes it really does work.

Word problems are a way of thinking and require you to translate a real word problem into mathematical terms.

Some math instructors go so far as to say that learning how to think mathematically is the main reason for teaching word problems.

So what do we mean by Practice regularly and systematically? Studying word problems and math in general requires a logical and mathematical frame of mind. The only way you can get this is by practicing regularly, which means everyday.

It is critical that you practice word problems everyday for the 5 days before the exam as a bare minimum.

If you practice and miss a day, you have lost the mathematical frame of mind and the benefit of your previous practice is pretty much gone. Anyone who has done any amount of math will agree – you have to practice everyday.

Everything is important. The other critical point about word problems is that all the information given in the problem has some purpose. There is no unnecessary information! Word problems are typically around 50 words in 1 to 3 sentences. If the sometimes complicated relationships are to be explained in that short an explanation, every word has to count. Make sure that you use every piece of information.

Here are 9 simple steps to help you resolve word problems.

Step 1 – Read through the problem at least three times. The first reading should be a quick scan, and the next two readings should be done slowly with a view to finding answers to these important questions:

What does the problem ask? (Usually located towards the end of the problem)

What does the problem imply? (This is usually a point you were asked to remember).

Mark all information, and underline all important words or phrases.

Step 2 – Try to make a pictorial representation of the problem such as a circle and an arrow to indicate travel. This makes the problem a bit more real and sensible to you.

A favorite word problem is something like, 1 train leaves Station A travelling at 100 km/hr and another train leaves Station B travelling at 60 km/hr. ...

Draw a line, the two stations, and the two trains at either end. This will help solidify the situation in your mind.

Step 3 – Use the information you have to make a table with a blank portion to indicate information you do not know.

Step 4 – Assign a single letter to represent each unknown data in your table. You can write down the unknown that each letter represents so that you do not make the error of assigning answers to the wrong unknown, because a word problem may have multiple unknowns and you will need to create equations for each unknown.

Step 5 – Translate the English terms in the word problem into a mathematical algebraic equation. Remember that the main problem with word problems is that they are not expressed in regular math equations. You ability to correctly identify the variables and translate the word problem into an equation determines your ability to solve the problem.

Step 6 – Check the equation to see if it looks like regular equations that you are used to seeing and whether it looks sensible. Does the equation appear to represent the information in the question? Take note that you may need to rewrite some formulas needed to solve the word problem equation. For example, word distance problems may need rewriting the distance formula, which is Distance = Time x Rate. If the word problem requires that you solve for time you will need to use Distance/Rate and Distance/Time to solve for Rate. If you understand the distance word problem you should be able to identify the variable you need to solve for.

Step 7 – Use algebra rules to solve the derived equation. Take note that the laws of equation demands that what is done on this side of the equation has to also be done on the other side. You have to solve the equation so that the unknown ends up alone on one side. Where there are multiple unknowns you will need to use elimination or substitution methods to resolve all the equations.

Step 8 – Check your final answers to see if they make sense with the information given in the problem. For example if the word problem involves a discount, the final price should be less or if a product was taxed then the final answer has to cost more.

Step 9 – Cross check your answers by placing the answer or answers in the first equation to replace the unknown or unknowns. If your answer is correct then both side of the equation must equate or equal. If your answer is not correct then you may have derived a wrong equation or solved the equation wrongly. Repeat the necessary steps to correct.

Types of Word Problems

Word problems can be classified into 12 types. Below are examples of each type with a complete solution. Some types of word problems can be solved quickly using multiple choice strategies and some can not. Always look for ways to estimate the answer and then eliminate choices.

1. Age

A girl is 10 years older than her brother. By next year, she will be twice the age of her brother. What are their ages now?

    a. 25, 15
    b. 19, 9
    c. 21, 11
    d. 29, 19

Solution: B

We will assume that the girl's age is "a" and her brother's is "b". This means that based on the information in the first sentence,
$a = 10 + b$

Next year, she will be twice her brother's age, which gives
$a + 1 = 2(b+1)$

We need to solve for one unknown factor and then use the answer to solve for the other. To do this we substitute the value of "a" from the first equation into the second equation. This gives

$10+b + 1 = 2b + 2$
$11 + b = 2b + 2$
$11 - 2 = 2b - b$
$b = 9$

$9 = b$ this means that her brother is 9 years old. Solving for the girl's age in the first equation gives $a = 10 + 9$. $a = 19$ the girl is aged 19. So, the girl is aged 19 and the boy is 9

2. Distance or speed

Two boats travel down a river towards the same destination, starting at the same time. One boat is traveling at 52 km/hr, and the other boat at 43 km/hr. How far apart will they be after 40 minutes?

   a. 46.67 km
   b. 19.23 km
   c. 6 km
   d. 14.39 km

Solution: C

After 40 minutes, the first boat will have traveled = 52 km/hr x 40 minutes/60 minutes = 34.66 km
After 40 minutes, the second boat will have traveled = 43 km/hr x 40/60 minutes = 28.66 km
Difference between the two boats will be 34.66 km – 28.66 km = 6 km.

Multiple Choice Strategy

First estimate the answer. The first boat is travelling 9 km. faster than the second, for 40 minutes, which is 2/3 of an hour. 2/3 of 9 = 6, as a rough guess of the distance apart.

Choices A, B and D can be eliminated right away.

3. Ratio

The instructions in a cookbook states that 700 grams of flour must be mixed in 100 ml of water, and 0.90 grams of salt added. A cook however has just 325 grams of flour. What is the quantity of water and salt that he should use?

   a. 0.41 grams and 46.4 ml
   b. 0.45 grams and 49.3 ml
   c. 0.39 grams and 39.8 ml
   d. 0.25 grams and 40.1 ml

Solution: A

The Cookbook states 700 grams of flour, but the cook only has 325. The first

step is to determine the percentage of flour he has 325/700 x 100 = 46.4%
That means that 46.4% of all other items must also be used.
46.4% of 100 = 46.4 ml of water
46.4% of 0.90 = 0.41 grams of salt.

Multiple Choice Strategy

The recipe calls for 700 grams of flour but the cook only has 325, which is just less than half, the quantity of water and salt are going to be about half.

Choices C and D can be eliminated right away. Choice B is very close so be careful. Looking closely at Choice B, it is exactly half, and since 325 is slightly less than half of 700, it can't be correct.

Choice A is correct.

4. Percent

An agent received $6,685 as his commission for selling a property. If his commission was 13% of the selling price, how much was the property?

   a. $68,825
   b. $121,850
   c. $49,025
   d. $51,423

Solution: D

Let's assume that the property price is x
That means from the information given, 13% of x = 6,685
Solve for x,
x = 6685 x 100/13 = $51,423

Multiple Choice Strategy

The commission,13%, is just over 10%, which is easier to work with. Round up $6685 to $6700, and multiple by 10 for an approximate answer. 10 X 6700 = $67,000. You can do this in your head. Choice B is much too big and can be eliminated. Choice C is too small and can be eliminated. Choices A and D are left and good possibilities.

Do the calculations to make the final choice.

5. Sales & Profit

A store owner buys merchandise for $21,045. He transports them for $3,905 and pays his staff $1,450 to stock the merchandise on his shelves. If he does not incur further costs, how much does he need to sell the items to make $5,000 profit?

    a. $32,500

    b. $29,350

    c. $32,400

    d. $31,400

Solution: D

Total cost of the items is $21,045 + $3,905 + $1,450 = $26,400
Total cost is now $26,400 + $5000 profit = $31,400

Multiple Choice Strategy

Round off and add the numbers up in your head quickly.
21,000 + 4,000 + 1500 = 26500. Add in 5000 profit for a total of 31500.

Choice B is too small and can be eliminated. Choice C and Choice A are too large and can be eliminated.

6. Tax/Income

A woman earns $42,000 per month and pays 5% tax on her monthly income. If the Government increases her monthly taxes by $1,500, what is her income after tax?

    a. $38,400

    b. $36,050

    c. $40,500

    d. $39, 500

Solution: A

Initial tax on income was 5/100 x 42,000 = $2,100
$1,500 was added to the tax to give $2,100 + 1,500 = $3,600
Income after tax left is $42,000 - $3,600 = $38,400

7. Interest

A man invests $3000 in a 2-year term deposit that pays 3% interest per year. How much will he have at the end of the 2-year term?

    a. $5,200

    b. $3,020

    c. $3,182.7

    d. $3,000

Solution: C

This is a compound interest problem. The funds are invested for 2 years and interest is paid yearly, so in the second year, he will earn interest on the interest paid in the first year.

3% interest in the first year = 3/100 x 3,000 = $90
At end of first year, total amount = 3,000 + 90 = $3,090
Second year = 3/100 x 3,090 = 92.7.
At end of second year, total amount = $3090 + $92.7 = $3,182.7

8. Averaging

The average weight of 10 books is 54 grams. 2 more books were added and the average weight became 55.4. If one of the 2 new books added weighed 62.8 g, what is the weight of the other?

    a. 44.7 g

    b. 67.4 g

    c. 62 g

    d. 52 g

Solution: C

Total weight of 10 books with average 54 grams will be=10×54=540 g
Total weight of 12 books with average 55.4 will be=55.4×12=664.8 g
So total weight of the remaining 2 will be= 664.8 – 540 = 124.8 g
If one weighs 62.8, the weight of the other will be= 124.8 g – 62.8 g = 62 g

Multiple Choice Strategy

Averaging problems can be estimated by looking at which direction the average goes. If additional items are added and the average goes up, the new items much be greater than the average. If the average goes down after new items are added, the new items must be less than the average.

Here, the average is 54 grams and 2 books are added which increases the average to 55.4, so the new books must weight more than 54 grams.

Choices A and D can be eliminated right away.

9. Probability

A bag contains 15 marbles of various colors. If 3 marbles are white, 5 are red and the rest are black, what is the probability of randomly picking out a black marble from the bag?

a. 7/15
b. 3/15
c. 1/5
d. 4/15

Solution: A

Total marbles = 15
Number of black marbles = 15 − (3 + 5) = 7
Probability of picking out a black marble = 7/15

10. Two Variables

A company paid a total of $2850 to book for 6 single rooms and 4 double rooms in a hotel for one night. Another company paid $3185 to book for 13 single rooms for one night in the same hotel. What is the cost for single and double rooms in that hotel?

a. single= $250 and double = $345
b. single= $254 and double = $350
c. single = $245 and double = $305
d. single = $245 and double = $345

Solution: D

We can determine the price of single rooms from the information given of the second company. 13 single rooms = 3185.

One single room = 3185 / 13 = 245
The first company paid for 6 single rooms at $245. 245 x 6 = $1470
Total amount paid for 4 double rooms by first company = $2850 - $1470 = $1380
Cost per double room = 1380 / 4 = $345

11. Geometry

The length of a rectangle is 5 in. more than its width. The perimeter of the rectangle is 26 in. What is the width and length of the rectangle?

    a. width = 6 inches, Length = 9 inches
    b. width = 4 inches, Length = 9 inches
    c. width =4 inches, Length = 5 inches
    d. width = 6 inches, Length = 11 inches

Solution: B

Formula for perimeter of a rectangle is 2(L + W)
p=26, so 2(L+W) = p
The length is 5 inches more than the width, so
2(w+5) + 2w = 26
2w + 10 + 2w = 26
2w + 2w = 26 - 10
4w = 16

W = 16/4 = 4 inches

L is 5 inches more than w, so L = 5 + 4 = 9 inches.

12. Totals and Fractions

A basket contains 125 oranges, mangos and apples. If 3/5 of the fruits in the basket are mangos and only 2/5 of the mangos are ripe, how many ripe mangos are there in the basket?

    a. 30
    b. 68
    c. 55
    d. 47

Solution: A
Number of mangos in the basket is 3/5 x 125 = 75
Number of ripe mangos = 2/5 x 75 = 30

Natural Science

This section contains a natural science self-assessment and tutorials. The Tutorials are designed to familiarize general principles and the Self-Assessment contains general questions similar to the science questions likely to be on the PSB exam, but are not intended to be identical to the exam questions. Many Universities recommend that students take an introductory science course before taking the PSB exam. The tutorials are *not* designed to be a complete science course, and it is assumed that students have some familiarity with natural sciences. If you do not understand parts of the tutorial, or find the tutorial difficult, it is recommended that you seek out additional instruction.

Tour of the PSB Science Content

Below is a detailed list of the science topics likely to appear on the PSB. Make sure that you understand these at the very minimum.

- Understand general human anatomy and physiology

- Biological classification

- Parts of a cell and functions

- Mitosis and Meiosis

- Photosynthesis and respiration

- DNA and RNA, including mutations and cell replication

- Basic Heredity (Mendel and Punnett squares)

- Chromosomes, genes and proteins

- Phenotypes and genotypes

- Basic chemical reactions such as oxidation/reduction and acid/base reactions

- Catalysts

- Chemical bonds

- Types of energy - Kinetic, potential, mechanical

- Atoms, protons, neutrons and electrons

- The Periodic Table

- States of matter - liquids, gases and solids

- Simple changes of state including evaporation, vaporization and condensation

- Understand scientific reasoning

- Identify steps in a scientific investigation

The questions below are not the same as you will find on the PSB - that would be too easy! And nobody knows what the questions will be and they change all the time. Mostly the changes consist of substituting new questions for old, but the changes also can be new question formats or styles, changes to the number of questions in each section, changes to the time limits for each section and combing sections. Below are general Science questions that cover the same areas as the PSB. So, while the format and exact wording of the questions may differ slightly, and changes from year to year, if you can answer the questions below, you will have no problem with the natural science section of the PSB.

Self Assessment

The purpose of the self-assessment is:

- Identify your strengths and weaknesses.

- Develop your personalized study plan (see Chapter 1)

- Get accustomed to the PSB format

- Extra practice – the self-assessment is a 3rd test!

- Provide a baseline score for preparing your study schedule.

Since this is a self-assessment, and depending on how confident you are with basic science, timing yourself is optional. Once complete, use the table below to assess you understanding of the content, and prepare your study schedule described in chapter 1.

80% - 100%	Excellent – you have mastered the content
60 – 79%	Good. You have a working knowledge. Even though you can just pass this section, you may want to review the Tutorials and do some extra practice to see if you can improve your mark.
40% - 59%	Below Average. You do not understand the problems. Review the tutorials, and retake this quiz again in a few days, before proceeding to the rest of the practice test questions.
Less than 40%	Poor. You have a very limited understanding of the reading comprehension problems. Please review the Tutorials, and retake this quiz again in a few days, before proceeding to the rest of the study guide.

Science Self Assessment Answer Sheet

1. (A) (B) (C) (D)   11. (A) (B) (C) (D)   21. (A) (B) (C) (D)

2. (A) (B) (C) (D)   12. (A) (B) (C) (D)   22. (A) (B) (C) (D)

3. (A) (B) (C) (D)   13. (A) (B) (C) (D)   23. (A) (B) (C) (D)

4. (A) (B) (C) (D)   14. (A) (B) (C) (D)   24. (A) (B) (C) (D)

5. (A) (B) (C) (D)   15. (A) (B) (C) (D)   25. (A) (B) (C) (D)

6. (A) (B) (C) (D)   16. (A) (B) (C) (D)   26. (A) (B) (C) (D)

7. (A) (B) (C) (D)   17. (A) (B) (C) (D)   27. (A) (B) (C) (D)

8. (A) (B) (C) (D)   18. (A) (B) (C) (D)   28. (A) (B) (C) (D)

9. (A) (B) (C) (D)   19. (A) (B) (C) (D)   29. (A) (B) (C) (D)

10. (A) (B) (C) (D)   20. (A) (B) (C) (D)   30. (A) (B) (C) (D)

1. Which system can be thought of as the blood distribution system?

    a. Digestive system.

    b. Musculoskeletal system.

    c. Endocrine system.

    d. Circulatory system

2. What are examples of nutrients circulated via the circulatory system?

    a. Citric acids

    b. Amino acids

    c. Proteins

    d. Nuclei

3. What is the primary purpose of the digestive system?

    a. To expel food and liquids from the body.

    b. To absorb oxygen from food.

    c. To help circulate blood throughout the body.

    d. To convert food into a form that can provide nourishment for the body.

4. Which element in the digestive process helps break down food?

    a. Digestive juices

    b. Proteins

    c. Amino acids

    d. Chromosomes

5. What is the respiratory system?

    a. The system that brings oxygen into the body and expels carbon dioxide from the body.

    b. The system that sends blood to and from the heart.

    c. The system which processes food that enters the body.

    d. The system which expels urine from the body.

6. Which, if any, of the following statements about the respiratory system are true?

a. The respiratory system consists of all the organs involved in breathing.

b. Organs included in the respiratory system are the nose, pharynx, larynx, trachea, bronchi and lungs.

c. The respiratory system conveys oxygen into our bodies and removes carbon dioxide from our bodies.

d. All of the Above.

7. Which of the following are an important component of the respiratory system?

a. The cornea

b. The lungs

c. The kidneys

d. The stomach

8. A _____ is a naturally occurring assemblage of plants and animals that occupy a common environment.

a. Society

b. Biosphere

c. Community

d. Population

9. Classification is a grouping of organisms based on similar

a. Traits and evolutionary histories

b. Traits and biological histories

c. Behaviors and evolutionary histories

d. Traits and evolutionary advancement

10. A method for categorizing organisms by their biological type is known as:

    a. Anatomical classification.

    b. Biological classification.

    c. Physical classification.

    d. Cellular classification.

11. When compared to homologous traits, "analogous" traits refer to ones that:

    a. Are similar but the similarity does not derive from a common ancestor.

    b. Are similar because they had the same parents.

    c. Are not similar and do not come from a common ancestor.

    d. Are completely equal.

12. Which, if any, of the following statements about mitosis are correct?

    a. Mitosis is the process of cell division by which identical daughter cells are produced.

    b. Following mitosis, new cells contain less DNA than did the original cells.

    c. During mitosis, the chromosome number is doubled.

    d. A and C are correct.

13. What is a nucleic acid that carries the genetic information in the cell and is capable of self-replication?

    a. RNA

    b. Triglyceride

    c. DNA

    d. DAR

14. The segment of a DNA molecule determining the amino acid sequence of protein is known as

    a. Operator gene

    b. Structural gene

    c. Regulator gene

    d. Modifier gene

15. Cells that line the inner or outer surfaces of organs or body cavities are often linked together by intimate physical connections. What are these connections?

    a. Separate desmosomes

    b. Ronofilaments

    c. Tight junctions

    d. Fascia adherenes

16. Genes control heredity in man and other organisms. These genes are

    a. A segment of RNA or DNA

    b. A bead like structure on the chromosomes

    c. A protein molecule

    d. A segment of RNA

17. Describe the systems in our bodies.

    a. Our bodies have 5 different systems, including circulatory, digestive, and lymphatic.

    b. Our bodies have 11 different systems, including circulatory, digestive, and heart.

    c. Our bodies have 11 different systems, including circulatory, digestive, and lymphatic.

    d. Our bodies have 12 different systems, including circulatory, bowel, and lymphatic.

18. Who was a 19th century scientist who outlined the original theory of inheritance?

    a. Albert Einstein

    b. Christian Doppler

    c. Gregor Mendel

    d. Charles Darwin

19. Describe the science of genetics.

    a. Is a branch of biology concerned with the study of heredity and variation.

    b. Attempts to explain how characteristics of living organisms are passed on from one generation to the next.

    c. Is a measure of the variety of the of the Earth's animal, plant, and microbial species.

    d. A and B

20. What is the overall measure of the variety of the Earth's animal, plant, and microbial species, of genetic differences within species, and of the ecosystems that support those species?

    a. Environment

    b. Bionetwork

    c. Ecology

    d. Biodiversity

21. In the periodic table of the elements, elements are arranged in order of their atomic _____, which is the number of _____ found in their nucleus.

    a. Mass, protons

    b. Number, neutrons

    c. Mass, neutrons

    d. Number, protons

22. Any physical manifestation that is part of the observable structure, function or behavior of a living organism is its _____.

    a. Genetic code

    b. Chromosome

    c. Genotype

    d. Phenotype

23. Protons, neutrons, and electrons differ in that:

a. Protons and neutrons form the nucleus of an atom, while electrons are found in

fixed energy levels around the nucleus of the atom.

b. Protons and neutrons are charged particles and electrons are neutral.

c. Protons and neutrons form fixed energy levels around the nucleus of the atom and electrons are located near the surface of the atom.

d. Protons, neutrons and electrons are charged particles.

24. What are considered to be the four fundamental forces of nature?

a. Gravity, electromagnetic force, weak nuclear force, and strong nuclear force

b. Gravity, electromagnetic force, negative nuclear force, and positive nuclear force

c. Polarity, electromagnetic force, weak nuclear force, and strong nuclear force

d. Gravity, chemical magnetic force, weak nuclear force, and strong nuclear force

25. Which of these statements about mechanical energy is/are true?

a. Mechanical energy is the energy that is possessed by an object due to its motion or due to its position.

b. Mechanical energy can be either kinetic energy (energy of motion) or potential energy (stored energy of position).

c. Objects have mechanical energy if they are in motion

d. All of the above.

26. Evaporation is:

a. A type of vaporization that occurs within the mass of a liquid

b. A type of vaporization that occurs from the surface of a liquid

c. A type of vaporization that occurs from the surface and within the mass of a liquid.

d. None of the above

27. Describe enzymes

a. Most enzymes are proteins that are selective catalysts

b. Enzymes are catalysts that accelerate metabolic reactions

c. Enzymes are chemical agents that assist metabolic reactions

d. Enzymes are biological agents that decrease the rate of reaction

28. In science, _____ is defined as a difference between the desired and actual performance or behavior of a system or object.

a. Accuracy

b. Uncertainty

c. Error

d. Mistake

29. When employing the scientific method of research, the researcher follows these steps:

a. Define the question, make observations, offer a possible explanation, perform an experiment, analyze data, draw conclusions.

b. Make observations, offer a possible explanation, define the question, perform an experiment, analyze, draw conclusions.

c. Perform an experiment, make observations, define the question, offer a possible explanation, analyze the data, draw conclusions.

d. Make observations, define the question, offer a possible explanation, perform an experiment, analyze data, draw conclusions.

30. What is the principle that generally advises choosing the competing hypothesis that makes the fewest new assumptions, when the hypotheses are equal in other respects.

a. Hickam's Dictum

b. Boyle's Law

c. Dalton's Law

d. Occam's Razor

Answer Key

1. D
The circulatory system can be thought of as the blood distribution system.

2. B
The circulatory system is a system that passes nutrients (such as amino acids, electrolytes and lymph), gases, hormones, blood cells, etc. to and from cells in the body to help fight diseases, help stabilize body temperature and pH.

3. D
The primary purpose of the digestive system is to convert food into a form that can provide nourishment for the body.

4. A
Digestive juices such as gastric acid are formed in the stomach. It has a pH of 1 to 2 and is composed of hydrochloric acid (HCl) (around 0.5%, or 5000 parts per million), and large quantities of potassium chloride (KCl) and sodium chloride (NaCl). The acid plays a key role in digestion of proteins, by activating digestive enzymes, and making ingested proteins unravel so that digestive enzymes can break down the long chains of amino acids.

5. A
The respiratory system is the anatomical system of an organism that introduces respiratory gases to the interior and performs gas exchange. The anatomical features of the respiratory system include airways, lungs, and the respiratory muscles. Molecules of oxygen and carbon dioxide are passively exchanged, by diffusion, between the gaseous external environment and the blood. This exchange process occurs in the alveolar region of the lungs.

6. D
All of the statements are true.

    a. The respiratory system consists of all the organs involved in breathing.

    b. Organs included in the respiratory system are the nose, pharynx, larynx, trachea, bronchi and lungs.

    c.The respiratory system conveys oxygen into our bodies and removes carbon dioxide from our bodies.

7. B
The Lungs are an important component of the respiratory system.

8. C

Communities are usually named after a dominant feature, such as characteristic plant species, e.g. pine.

9. A

Classification is a grouping of organisms based on similar traits and evolutionary histories.

Note: Taxonomy and systematics are the two sciences that attempt to classify living things. In taxonomy, organisms are assigned to groups based on their characteristics. In modern systematics, the placement of organisms into groups is based on evolutionary relationships.

10. B

Biological classification. Classification is more a matter of convenience; in reality, there are many times when the various classifications tend to blur into each other.

11 A

Analogous traits are similar but the similarity does not derive from a common ancestor.

12. A and C are correct.

  a. Mitosis is the process of cell division by which identical daughter cells are produced.

  c. During mitosis, the chromosome number is doubled.

13. C

DNA is a nucleic acid that carries the genetic information in the cell and is capable of self-replication.

14. B

A structural gene is the segment of a DNA molecule determining the amino acid sequence of protein. DNA is a nucleic acid that contains the genetic instructions used in the development and functioning of all known living organisms (except for RNA viruses). The DNA segments that carry this genetic information are called genes but other DNA sequences have structural purposes or are involved in regulating the use of this genetic information. Along with RNA and proteins DNA is one of the three major macromolecules that are essential for all known forms of life. [4]

15. C

Tight junctions or zonula occludens are the closely associated areas of two cells whose membranes join forming a virtually impermeable barrier to fluid. It is a type of junctional complex present only in vertebrates. The corresponding junctions that occur in invertebrates are septate junctions. [5]

16. A

Genes are made from a long molecule called DNA which is copied and inherited across generations. DNA is made of simple units that line up in a particular order within this large molecule. The order of these units carries genetic information similar to how the order of letters on a page carries information. The language used by DNA is called the genetic code which lets organisms read the information in the genes. This information is the instructions for constructing and operating a living organism.

17. C

Our bodies have 11 different systems, including circulatory, digestive, and lymphatic.

Note: Other systems include the endocrine, immune, muscular, nervous, reproductive, respiratory, skeletal, and urinary systems.

18. C

Gregor Mendel was a 19th century scientist who outlined the original theory of inheritance.

19. D

a. Is a branch of biology concerned with the study of heredity and variation.

b. Attempts to explain how characteristics of living organisms are passed on from one generation to the next.

20. D

Biodiversity is an overall measure of the variety of the Earth's animal, plant, and microbial species, of genetic differences within species, and of the ecosystems that support those species.

Note: In the 20th century, the destruction of the rainforests and the spread of agriculture is believed to have resulted in the most severe and rapid loss of diversity in the history of the planet.

21. D

In the periodic table of the elements, elements are arranged in order of their atomic number, which is the number of protons found in their nucleus.

22. D

Any physical manifestation that is part of the observable structure, function or behavior of a living organism is its phenotype.

23. A

Protons and neutrons form the nucleus of an atom, while electrons are found infixed energy levels around the nucleus of the atom.

24. A

The four fundamental forces of nature are, gravity, electromagnetic force, weak nuclear force, and strong nuclear force.

Note: Electromagnetic force is more commonly known as electricity.

25. D

All the statements are true.

> a. Mechanical energy is the energy that is possessed by an object due to its motion or due to its position.
>
> b. Mechanical energy can be either kinetic energy (energy of motion) or potential energy (stored energy of position).
>
> c. Objects have mechanical energy if they are in motion

Note: Objects also have mechanical energy if they are at some position relative to a zero potential energy position, for example, a brick held at a vertical position above the ground. [6]

26. B

Evaporation is a type of vaporization of a liquid that only occurs on the surface of a liquid. The other type of vaporization is boiling, which, instead, occurs within the entire mass of the liquid.

27. A

Most enzymes are proteins that are selective catalysts

28. C

In science, Error is a difference between the desired and actual performance or behavior of a system or object.

29. A

When employing the scientific method of research, the researcher follows these steps: define the question, make observations, offer a possible explanation, perform an experiment, analyze data, draw conclusions.

30. D
Occam's Razor is a principle that generally advises choosing the competing hypothesis that makes the fewest new assumptions, when the hypotheses are equal in other respects.

Scientific Method

The scientific method is a set of steps that allow people who ask "how" and "why" questions about the world to go about finding valid answers that accurately reflect reality.

Were it not for the scientific method, people would have no valid method for drawing quantifiable and accurate information about the world.

There are four primary steps to the scientific method:

1. Analyzing an aspect of reality and asking "how" or "why" it works or exists
2. Forming a hypothesis that explains "how" or "why"
3. Making a prediction about the sort of things that would happen if the hypothesis were true
4. Performing an experiment to test your prediction.

These steps vary somewhat depending on the field of science you happen to be studying. (In astronomy, for instance, experiments are generally eschewed in favor of observational evidence confirming that predictions are true.) But for the most part, this is the model scientists follow.

Observation and Analysis

The first step in the scientific method requires you to determine what it is about reality that you want to explore.

You might notice that your friends who eat regular servings of fruits and vegetables are healthier and more athletic than your friends who live off red meat and meals covered in cheese and gravy. This is an observation and, noting it, you are likely to ask yourself "why" it seems to be true. At this stage of the scientific method, scientists will often do research to see if anyone else has explored similar observations and analyze what other people's findings have been. This is an important step not only because it can show you what others have found to be true about their observation, but because it can show what others have found to be false, which can be equally as valuable.

Hypothesis

After making your observation and doing some research, you can form your hypothesis. A hypothesis is an idea you formulate based on the evidence you have already gathered about "how" your observation relates to reality.

Using the example of your friends' diets, you may have found research discussing vitamin levels in fruits and vegetables and how certain vitamins will affect a person's health and athleticism. This research may lead you to hypothesize that the foods your healthy friends are eating contain specific types of vitamins, and it is the vitamins making them healthy. Just as importantly, however, is applying research that shows hypotheses that were later proven wrong. Scientists need to know this information, too, as it can help keep them from making errors in their thinking. For instance, you could come across a research paper in which someone hypothesized that the sugars in fruits and vegetables gave people more energy, which then helped them be more athletic. If the paper were to go onto explain that no such link was found, and that the protein and carbohydrates in meat and gravy contained far more energy than the sugar, you would know that this hypothesis was wrong and that there was no need for you to waste time exploring it.

Prediction

The third step in the scientific method is making a prediction based on your hypothesis.

Forming predictions is vital to the scientific method because if your prediction turns out to be correct, it will demonstrate that your hypothesis can accurately explain some aspect of the world. This is important because one aspect of the scientific method is its ability to prove objectively that your way of understanding the world is valid. We can take the simple example of a car that will not start. If you notice the fuel gauge is pointing towards empty, you can announce your prediction to the other passengers that a careful test of the gas tank will show the car has no fuel. While this seems obvious, it is still important to note since a prediction like this is the only way to really *prove* to your friends that you understand how a fuel gauge works and what it means.

In the same way a prediction made by a hypothesis is the only way to really show that it represents reality. For instance, based on your vitamin hypothesis you may predict people can be healthy and athletic while eating whatever they want as long as they take vitamin supplements. If this prediction ends being true, it will show that it is in fact the vitamins, and only the vitamins, in fruits and vegetables that make people healthy and athletic. It will prove that your hypothesis shows how vitamins work.

Experiment

The final step is to perform an experiment that tests your prediction.

You may decide to separate your healthy friends into three groups, give one group vitamin supplements and prohibit them from eating vegetables, give another fake supplements and prohibit them from eating vegetables and have the third act normally as the control group. It is always important to have a control group so you have someone acting "normally" to compare your results against. If this experiment shows the real supplement group and the control group maintaining the same level of health and athleticism while the fake supplement group grows weak and sickly, you will know your hypothesis is true. If, on the other hand, you get unexpected results, you will need to go back to step one, analyze your results, make new observations and try again with a different hypothesis.

Any hypothesis that cannot be confirmed with experiment (or in the case of fields such as astronomy, with observation) cannot be considered true and must be altered or abandoned. It is in this stage where scientists—being humans, with human beliefs and prejudices—are most likely to abandon the scientific method. If an experiment or observation gives a scientist results that he or she does not like, the scientist may be inclined to ignore the results rather than reexamine the hypothesis. This was the case for nearly a thousand years in astronomy with astronomers attempting to form accurate models of the solar system based on circular orbits of the planets and on Earth being in the center. For philosophical reasons it was believed that circles were "perfect" and that the Earth was "important," so no model that had the correct elliptical orbits or the sun properly in the center was accepted until the 16th century, even though those models more accurately described all astronomers' observations.

Biology

Biology is a natural science concerned with the study of life and living organisms, including their structure, function, growth, origin, evolution, distribution, and taxonomy.

Biology is a vast subject containing many subdivisions, topics, and disciplines. Among the most important topics are five unifying principles that can be said to be the fundamental axioms of modern biology:

- Cells are the basic unit of life

- New species and inherited traits are the product of evolution

- Genes are the basic unit of heredity

- An organism regulates its internal environment to maintain a stable and constant condition

- Living organisms consume and transform energy.

Sub-disciplines of biology are recognized by the scale at which organisms are studied and the methods used to study them: biochemistry examines the rudimentary chemistry of life; molecular biology studies the complex interactions of systems of biological molecules; cellular biology examines the basic building block of all life, the cell; physiology examines the physical and chemical functions of the tissues, organs, and organ systems of an organism; and ecology examines how various organisms interact and associate with their environment.[7]

Cell Biology

Cell biology (formerly cytology, from the Greek kytos, "contain") is a scientific discipline that studies cells – their physiological properties, their structure, the organelles they contain, interactions with their environment, their life cycle, division and death.

This is done both on a microscopic and molecular level. Cell biology research encompasses both the great diversity of single-celled organisms like bacteria and protozoa, as well as the many specialized cells in multicellular organisms such as humans.

Knowing the components of cells and how cells work is fundamental to all biological sciences.

Appreciating the similarities and differences between cell types is particularly important to the fields of cell and molecular biology as well as to biomedical fields such as cancer research and developmental biology. These fundamental similarities and differences provide a unifying theme, sometimes allowing the principles learned from studying one cell type to be extrapolated and generalized to other cell types. Therefore, research in cell biology is closely related to genetics, biochemistry, molecular biology, immunology, and developmental biology.

Each type of protein is usually sent to a particular part of the cell.

An important part of cell biology is the investigation of molecular mechanisms by which proteins are moved to different places inside cells or secreted from cells.

Processes – Movement of Proteins

Most proteins are synthesized by ribosomes in the rough endoplasmic reticulum.

Ribosomes contain the nucleic acid RNA, which assembles and joins amino acids to make proteins. They can be found alone or in groups within the cytoplasm as well as on the RER.

This process is known as protein biosynthesis.

Biosynthesis (also called biogenesis) is an enzyme-catalyzed process in cells of living organisms by which substrates are converted to more complex products (also simply known as protein translation). Some proteins, such as those to be incorporated in membranes (known as membrane proteins), are transported into the "rough" endoplasmic reticulum (ER) during synthesis. This process can be followed by transportation and processing in the Golgi apparatus.

The Golgi apparatus is a large organelle that processes proteins and prepares them for use both inside and outside the cell.

The Golgi apparatus is somewhat like a post office. It receives items (proteins from the ER), packages and labels them, and then sends them on to their destinations (to different parts of the cell or to the cell membrane for transport out of the cell). From the Golgi, membrane proteins can move to the plasma membrane, to other sub-cellular compartments, or they can be secreted from the cell.

The ER and Golgi can be thought of as the "membrane protein synthesis compartment" and the "membrane protein processing compartment", respectively.

There is a semi-constant flux of proteins through these compartments. ER and Golgi-resident proteins associate with other proteins but remain in their respective compartments. Other proteins "flow" through the ER and Golgi to the plasma membrane. Motor proteins transport membrane protein-containing vesicles along cytoskeletal tracks to distant parts of cells such as axon terminals.

Some proteins that are made in the cytoplasm contain structural features that target them for transport into mitochondria or the nucleus.

Some mitochondrial proteins are made inside mitochondria and are coded for by mitochondrial DNA. In plants, chloroplasts also make some cell proteins.

Extracellular and cell surface proteins destined to be degraded can move back into intracellular compartments upon being incorporated into endocytosed vesicles some of which fuse with lysosomes where the proteins are broken down to their individual amino acids. The degradation of some membrane proteins begins while still at the cell surface when they are separated by secretases. Proteins that function in the cytoplasm are often degraded by proteasomes.

Other cellular processes

Active and Passive transport - Movement of molecules into and out of cells.
Autophagy - The process whereby cells "eat" their own internal components or microbial invaders.
Adhesion - Holding together cells and tissues.
Reproduction - Made possible by the combination of sperm made in the testiculi (contained in some male cells' nuclei) and the egg made in the ovary (contained in the nucleus of a female cell). When the sperm breaks through the hard outer shell of the egg a new cell embryo is formed, which, in humans, grows to full size in 9 months.
Cell movement - Chemotaxis, Contraction, cilia and flagella.
Cell signalling - Regulation of cell behavior by signals from outside.
DNA repair and Cell death
Metabolism - Glycolysis, respiration, Photosynthesis
Transcription and mRNA splicing - gene expression.

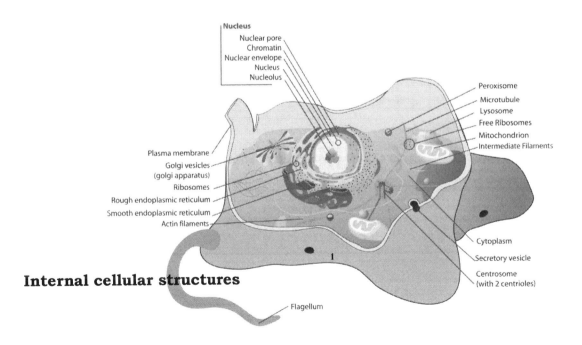

Internal cellular structures

Chloroplast - key organelle for photosynthesis (only found in plant cells)

Cilia - motile microtubule-containing structures of eukaryotes

Cytoplasm - contents of the main fluid-filled space inside cells

Cytoskeleton - protein filaments inside cells

Endoplasmic reticulum - major site of membrane protein synthesis

Flagella - motile structures of bacteria, archaea and eukaryotes

Golgi apparatus - site of protein glycosylation in the endomembrane system

Lipid bilayer - fundamental organizational structure of cell membranes

Lysosome - break down cellular waste products and debris into simple compounds (only found in animal cells)

Membrane lipid and protein barrier

Mitochondrion - major energy-producing organelle by releasing it in the form of ATP

Nucleus - holds most of the DNA of eukaryotic cells and controls all cellular activities

Organelle - term used for major subcellular structures

Ribosome - RNA and protein complex required for protein synthesis in cells

Vesicle - small membrane-bounded spheres inside cells

Chromosomes, genes, proteins, RNA and DNA

The concepts of genes, chromosomes, proteins, RNA and DNA are all interrelated genetic terms. Chromosomes are made up of genes, the DNA contains the chromosomes and the RNA interprets and implements the information in the RNA. Here is a break down of each of them.

Proteins

Proteins are biological molecules that are made up of a chain or chains of amino acids. Proteins play many very vital roles in living organisms. Protein is essential for the performance of many bodily functions such as replicating DNA, transporting nutrients and molecules within the body, responding to stimuli, and acting as a catalyst for metabolic reactions within the living organism, among other things. There are different types of proteins and they play various roles. The difference in proteins would be determined by their unique arrangement or sequence of amino acids.

Genes

A gene is the molecular hereditary unity of an organism and a small part of the chromosome. It is the term used to describe a portion of RNA or DNA code that performs a particular function in the organism. Genes are essential to life because they specify the functions of all proteins and RNA chains. Genes contain the information to maintain and build the cells in the organism and also contain genetic information that would be passed onto the offspring.

Genes hold the information for biological traits and functions some of which can clearly be seen and some of which are hidden. For example, the information contained in specific genes determines factors such as eye color, hair color, number of limbs, height and so on. Some traits such as blood type and the thousands of metabolic reactions and biochemical process that take place in the body to sustain life are defined unseen by the genes.

A gene is set of basic instruction embedded on a sequence of nucleic acids. The gene is a locatable region of the DNA genome sequence that correspond to a unit of inheritance and associated with a particular body function or set of functions.

Chromosomes

The chromosome is a piece of the DNA containing several genes. The chromosome is an organized part of the DNA. It is a single piece of coiled DNA. The chromosome contains several genes, DNA-bound proteins, nucleotide sequences and regulatory elements. The DNA-bound proteins help to hold the DNA together and regulate its functions.

Since the chromosomes contain the genes, they contain almost all the genetic information of the organism. Chromosomes differ from one organism to another. The DNA molecule could be linear or circular. The chromosome can contain from 100,000 to over 3 million nucleotides in one long chain depending on the organism. Cells with defined nuclei (eukaryotic cells) usually have large linear shaped chromosomes. Cells without clearly defined nuclei (prokaryotic cells) usually have smaller sized circular chromosomes.

Chromosomes are essential in the process of cell division. In mitosis cell division, the chromosomes have to be replicated and then divided among the two resulting daughter cells. This ensures that the resulting two daughter cells are genetically identical to the original mother cell.

DNA

DNA or Deoxyribonucleic acid is an essential component of life. It has been described as the blueprint of a living organism. It contains vital genetic information and instructions that are required for the proper functioning and development of all types and forms of living organisms and even viruses. DNA, proteins and RNA are the three most important macro-molecules that are essential for any form of life.

The genetic information contained in the DNA is encoded as a sequence of nucleotides known as G, A, and C. With G being guanine, A, adenine, T, thymine and C cytosine. These nucleotides are arranged as DNA molecules in a double-stranded helix. The strands run in opposite directions and are thus anti-parallel. The DNA contains long structures known as chromosomes.

RNA

RNA or Ribonucleic acids are large biological molecules that perform the important roles of decoding, coding, regulating and expressing the genes and the information contained within them. RNA, DNA and proteins are three essential components for all form of life. The RNA is also composed of nucleotides, but unlike the DNA that is double stranded, the RNA is single stranded.

In organisms, some RNA components serve as messengers to convey genetic information to direct the synthesis or use of specific proteins for specific purposes. It can thus be said that RNA is essential for the proper carrying out of the information contained in the DNA genes. RNA plays important roles within the cell such as helping to catalyze biological reactions sense and communicate cellular signals and control gene expressions. RNA is also essential for protein synthesis.

Mitosis and Meiosis

Meiosis and mitosis are two types of cellular division and they play a very important role in cell reproduction and the maintenance of tissues.

The cell is the basic functional unit of living organisms. It is made up of a collection of organelles and other cell matter dispersed within the cell membrane. For new cells to form, existing cells divide through the process of meiosis or mitosis, depending on the type of cell and reason for division.

Mitosis refers to the division of a cell into two identical cells.

The original cell goes through a process of duplication of its genetic material and then equally divides its contents into two new daughter cells.

The process of mitosis goes through several stages until the two cells segregate to form two distinct but genetically identical cells.

Mitosis cell division

During mitosis the cell divides its nucleus and then separates its organelles and chromosomes into two identical parts. The mother cell then divides into two genetically identical cells with equal parts of the cellular contents. The nuclei, cell membrane, organelles and cytoplasm of the cell would be shared between the two new cells.

Mitosis cell division is a complex and fast process. The process takes place in stages with each stage comprising of a set of activities that leads to the next set. The stages of mitosis are Prophase, Prometaphase, Metaphase, Anaphase and Telophase. Mitosis occurs in some unicellular organisms and within animal and human cells. Unicellular organisms use mitosis to reproduce their like and within animal and humans, mitosis is used to replace cells and repair tissues.

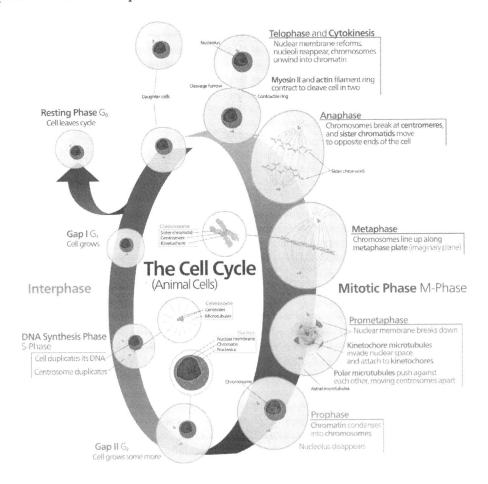

Meiosis

Meiosis occurs when one cells from the male and female combines or fuses together to form one diploid cell, which then splits to form four haploid cells.

The diploid cell contains copies of the chromosome and genetic information from both parents. The resulting four haploid cells will contain a copy of each chromosome.

Each chromosome in the four cells will contain a unique blend of the paternal and maternal genetic information, which makes it possible for the offspring to share some genetic resemblance to both parents while remaining genetically distinct from both of them. This nature of meiosis cell division is what accounts for the genetic diversity that is available today as each offspring DNA is a unique blend of its maternal and paternal genetic DNA.

Mitosis and meiosis have some similarities in that they are both types of cell division among living organisms.

There is however still some differences among them. For example, mitosis occurs within a cell with no interactions with other cells. The individual cell simply divides and produces two genetically identical cells. With meiosis, the process involves two cells from both the male and female in a form sexual reproduction. The resultant cells are four cells that are genetically different from their parents. The process of meiosis was discovered by Oscar Hertwig and Mitosis was discovered by Walther Flemming.

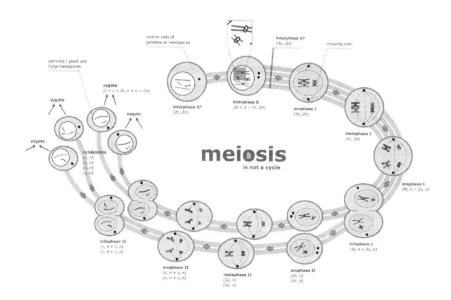

Phenotypes and Genotypes

The terms "phenotype" and "genotype" were first introduced in 1911 by Wilhelm Johannsen.

The term genotype refers to the genes of an organism that contains its complete hereditary information.

Phenotype refers to the actual observed properties of the organism.

Phenotypes deal with morphology, behavior and development. The distinction between genotypes and phenotypes is a very important fundamental aspect in the study of hereditary traits.

To explain the differences between the two concepts, one may look at genotypes as the inherited information about an organism. It is the genetic makeup of the traits, features and characteristics of the organism. Phenotype on the other hand defines the way that the information as spelled out by the genes is represented. Phenotype deals with the actual observable development and behavior.

A small or even minute difference in the genes of two organisms would mean that the two organisms have different genotypes.

Genes are hereditary and the genetic information contained is passed down from parents under control of specific molecular mechanisms. The genes or genetic information therein contained would affect or control the representation of the phenotype.

The genes define the trait or feature of the organism while the phenotype is the observable demonstration or expression of that trait. For example, if a mouse has a white color, it can be said that the genes defines that the mouse would be white and the phenotype is the white color that is observable. The genotype determines the phenotype, but the phenotype is also affected by external factors such as environmental factors.

A set of genotypes mapped to a set of phenotypes are referred to as a genotype-phenotype map.

The genotype is the largest influencer of an organism's phenotype, but is not the only influencing factor. That is why two identical twins that share the same genotype would still not have the same phenotypes. They may share identical genomes and their phenotype may even be quit similar, but it cannot be the same. That is why parents and close fiends would always be able to tell them apart. This is because their phenotype or the representation or expression of their genetic makeup as contained in their genotype would not be the same.

The term phenotype plasticity is used to describe the extent to which the genotype of an organism determines its phenotype.

An organism with weak or little phenotype plasticity would be highly determined more by its genotype and less by environmental factors.

An organism with high phenotype plasticity would have its phenotype more affected by environmental factors than by its genotype. A good example of an organism with high plasticity whose phenotype is more dependant on its environment than its genotype is the larval newt. The larvae would grow larger sized tails and heads relative to their body size when it notices the presence of their natural predators, i.e., the dragonfly.

Phenotype canalization is a term used to describe the extent that an organism's phenotype can be used to draw conclusions about the organism's genotype.

An organism with a canalized phenotype would be rarely affected by changes in its genotypes. If canalization is absent, very minor changes in the genome would result in immediate changes in the resulting phenotype.

Heredity: Genes and Mutation

All of the genetic material that tells our cells what jobs they hold is stored in our DNA (deoxyribonucleic acid). When complex creatures such as humans reproduce, our DNA is copied and combined with our mate's DNA to create a new genetic sequence for our offspring.

This information is stored in our genes and encoded in DNA base pairs through different combinations of the chemical groupings adenine and thymine (represented by A and T) and guanine and cytosine (represented by G and C). Each gene covers a small portion of our DNA and is responsible for creating the protein that section of DNA holds instructions for.

Genes contain two alleles, one from each of our parents. When we reproduce we will transfer one, and only one, of each allele to our children.

Alleles can be either dominant or recessive, and by combining the pairs of alleles we get from our parents, we can determine what our genes say we should be like. This genetic description of ourselves is known as our genotype. Genotype is our exact genetic makeup, and it determines our physical characteristics such as basic hair, eye and skin color. Related to the genotype is our phenotype, which describes the characteristics we display when our genes interact with the environment. For example, skin color is determined by a person's genotype, but the effect the sun has on skin—does the person tan, freckle, bun or even come away without any noticeable effect at all?—is an expression of phenotype.

Under normal circumstances people's genes will transfer directly from their parents following Mendel's Laws of Inheritance. Errors are common though.

DNA reproduction, however, is not necessarily a flawless process. Errors can develop either at random or due to outside influences such as radiation or chemicals in the environment. These errors, when related to heredity are called de novo mutations; they occur during embryonic development. Some mutations have no effect at all on the person's genetic makeup, but others can alter the way genes express themselves. Whether this is a good thing or not depends entirely on what genes are altered in what ways. Some mutations can cause children to be born sick or to have a higher susceptibility to disease by changing the types of proteins that their genes produce, or even by stopping certain proteins from being produced all together. Others, though, can be an improvement to the child's genetic structure. It is important to remember that the entire process of evolution is based on how random mutations throughout history have affected an individual's ability to interact with the environment.

Several notable examples of beneficial mutations stemming from natural selection can be seen in bubonic plague resistant European populations and malaria resistant African populations.

Both groups have genes built from specific alleles that create disease blocking proteins. (The CCR5 protein in people of European descent blocks the plague—and HIV sometimes—and the sickle cell protein in people of African descent blocks malaria.) These genes are widespread throughout their respective populations as a result of natural selection, which killed those who lived in these groups' ancestral regions but who did not possess the mutation. Had these diseases never existed, the mutations would have been considered neutral, providing no benefit yet causing no harm.

There are several ways that errors in DNA reproduction can cause mutations.

Chemicals can be inserted into, or deleted from base pairs, causing the chemical composition of the pairs to change and, thus, changing the alleles of the gene represented by those pairs. A portion of the DNA strand may also duplicate itself, or it may shift itself, causing the half of the base pair on one side of the DNA strand to link to the wrong half on the other side.

Heredity: Mendelian Inheritance

The father of genetics was a 19th century Austrian monk named Gregor Johann Mendel who became famous for his work crossbreeding peas in the garden of his monastery.

Aside from his life as a monk, Mendel was a highly educated physicist, studying first at the University of Olomouc (in the modern day Czech Republic) and later at the University of Vienna.

Mendel's work with peas revolutionized the scientific understanding of heredity and yielded two important laws: the Law of Segregation and the Law of Independent Assortment. To better understand these laws, however, we first need to look at the work of another geneticist, Reginald Punnett.

In 1900 while Punnett was doing his graduate work at the University of Cambridge in England, Gregor Mendel's work on genetics, which did not receive much attention during his lifetime, was being rediscovered. Punnett became an early follower of Mendelian genetics and developed the Punnett square as a means to organize the assortment of inherited alleles as Mendel described them. A Punnett square is simply a box with several squares drawn inside it and with the allele for a particular gene from each parent listed on either the top or the side. Each square shows a possible genotype (or set of alleles that define the gene) that can be inherited by the offspring of those parents. We will see Punnett squares as we explain Mendel's laws.

Law of Segregation

Mendel's Law of Segregation says that only half of the alleles of each parent's genes are transferred to their offspring, with the other half coming from the other parent.

Each gene contains two alleles. For instance a gene for trait 'A' could contain the alleles AA, Aa or aa, with the 'A' being the dominant form of the allele and 'a' being the recessive form. (Offspring with one or more dominant alleles exhibit the trait; offspring with only recessive forms do not.) The Law of Segregation says that one allele will come from one parent, and one will come from the other, and it is the parent's combined genetic makeup (rather than one parents particular genotype) that will determine the genes of their offspring.

Mendel also showed that the probability a certain trait would spread from parents to children was 3:1, provided that both parents had one dominant and one recessive form of the gene, also known has having heterozygous alleles. (Having two of the same alleles—AA or aa—is homozygous.)

Punnett squares

The Punnett square below represents the possible children born to two parents with Aa alleles expressing the 'A' gene.

	A	a
A	**AA**	**Aa**
a	**Aa**	aa

The three genes in bold, with at least one capital letter (AA, Aa and the other Aa), represent cases in which the presence of at least one dominant allele will cause the trait to manifest in the offspring. The remaining one (aa) represents the one case where the child does not manifest the trait even though both his or her parents do. (This could be the one brunette in a family of redheads, for instance.) Provided both parents have one dominant and one recessive allele, the distribution will always be 3:1.

Law of Independent Assortment

Mendel's second law, the Law of Independent Assortment, shows that the alleles of multiple genes will mix independently.

When two separate genotypes are tracked, the genes will produce 16 separate possible combinations spread out in a 9:3:3:1 ratio. This is also known as a dihybrid cross, while dealing with a single set of alleles is a monohybrid cross.

We can demonstrate this by assuming that we have a male and a female each with heterozygous alleles making them blond and tall. We can represent this with the genotypes BbTt in each. We should also assume that a 'bb' genotype would give someone brown hair and 'tt' would make them short. Since the Law of Independent Assortment says that each allele will mix independently, we end with four combinations of genotype that each parent can pass on: BT, Bt, bT and bt. These can then be mapped in a slightly larger Punnett square that looks like this:

	BT	Bt	bT	bt
BT	**BBTT**	**BBTt**	**BbTT**	**BbTt**
Bt	**BBTt**	**BBtt**	**BbTt**	**Bbtt**
bT	**BbTT**	**BbTt**	*bbTT*	*bbTt*
bt	**BbTt**	**Bbtt**	*bbTt*	bbtt

This is the distribution of the tall, blond couple's possible children. Nine would also be tall and blond, three would be short and blond, three would be tall and brunette, and one would be short and brunette. This perfectly follows the 9:3:3:1 ratio set out by Mendel.

Classification

Classification

Taxonomic classification is the primary method of organizing the Earth's biology.
Taxonomy means,

1. The classification of organisms in an ordered system that indicates natural relationships.
2. The science, laws, or principles of classification

The earliest form of classification that bears any resemblance to the current system can be traced back to ancient Greece with Aristotle's organization of animals based on reproduction.

The classification into kingdoms (animal, mineral and vegetable) was developed by Carolus Linnaeus.

The true father of modern taxonomical classification, however, is Carolus Linnaeus, who in the early 18th century developed a system of kingdoms that separated life into the categories animal, mineral and vegetable. Although Linnaeus's work lacked what would today be considered essential technologies (such as microscopes capable of imaging bacteria) and theories (such as evolution), much of his system has survived in modern classification.

Charles Darwin's theory of evolution was an important factor in taxonomic classification.

With Charles Darwin's publication of On the Origin of Species in 1859 the evolutionary process became a major factor in taxonomic classification. For the first time biology could be classified by grouping the direct descendents of common ancestors rather than just grouping creatures with similar characteristics.

The main classifications are, domain, kingdom, phylum, class, order, family, genus and species.

Today, most scientists accept a hierarchical structuring of biology that goes from general, or large, to specific: domain, kingdom, phylum, class, order, family, genus and species. (There are sometimes smaller subcategories such as superfamily, subfamily, tribe and subspecies listed, but these are the primary eight categories.) Domain is the newest of these and is split into three primary groups: Bacteria, Archaea and Eukarya. Each of these domains is split again with Bacteria splitting into the Kingdom Bacteria, Archaea splitting into the Kingdom Archaea and Eukarya splitting into the four kingdoms of Protista, Plantae, Fungi and finally our kingdom, Animalia. The Domain Eukarya splits so many times because eukaryotic cells are highly complex, containing such important features as cell walls and nuclei. As a result of this complexity, eukaryotic cells have gone through a much more diverse evolutionary process than prokaryotic cells such as bacteria and archaea, and thus Eukarya make up all complex life on Earth.

Rank	Fruit fly	Human	Pea	*E. coli*
Domain	Eukarya	Eukarya	Eukarya	Bacteria
Kingdom	Animalia	Animalia	Plantae	Bacteria
Phylum or **Division**	Arthropoda	Chordata	Magnoliophyta	
Subphylum or subdivision	Hexapoda	Vertebrata		
Class	Insecta	Mammalia	Magnoliopsida	
Subclass	Pterygota	Theria	Rosidae	
Order	Diptera	Primates	Fabales	
Suborder	Brachycera		Fabineae	
Family	Drosophilidae	Hominidae	Fabaceae	
Subfamily	Drosophilinae	Homininae	Faboideae	
Genus	*Drosophila*	*Homo*	*Pisum*	*Escherichia*
Species	*D. melanogaster*	*H. sapiens*	*P. sativum*	*E. coli*

8

Each Kingdom has a huge number of organisms. Bacteria and Archaea (single celled organisms).

Within each of the kingdoms the number of creatures is far too many to list. It is estimated that there could be as many as 100 million different species on Earth, although nowhere near that many have been physically catalogued. Of these, the majority are Bacteria and Archaea.

Another Example - Homo Sapiens

Since there is no way to list all the different subdivisions of life on Earth here, we might as well focus on one specific animal: us, Homo sapiens. We are members of the Domain Eukarya, the Kingdom Animalia, the Phylum Chordata, the Class Mammalia, the Order Primates, the Family Hominidae, the Genus Homo, the Species Homo sapiens and finally the Subspecies Homo sapiens sapiens. This classification is able to demonstrate our exact biological position in relation to life on Earth.

One important thing, a system like this tells us is that Homo, which is Latin for "human," is not actually our species, but our genus. This is an easy fact to forget since we are currently the only member of our genus not yet extinct. But anthropologically speaking there have been many humans including Homo habilis, Homo erectus and Homo neanderthalensis.

Taxonomical classification is an evolutionary map

Furthermore, the taxonomical classification system can be seen as a map of evolution on the planet. Plants, animals and bacteria can be traced back to common ancestors and newly discovered species can be classified in relation to their ancestors, descendants and cousins. The Genus Homo, for instance, is a direct offshoot of the Tribe Hominini. (A tribe is a subcategory of the category of family, which here is Hominidae.) Another genus that falls under the Tribe Hominini is Pan, which houses the species Chimpanzee. This shows us that until relatively recently in the history of life, Homo sapiens and Chimpanzees were the same creature, and that Chimpanzees only split off just before Homo sapiens became fully human.

Chemistry

Chemistry is the science of matter, especially its chemical reactions, but also its composition, structure and properties. Chemistry is concerned with atoms and their interactions with other atoms, and particularly with the properties of chemical bonds.

Chemistry is sometimes called "the central science" because it connects physics with other natural sciences such as geology and biology. Chemistry is a branch of physical science but distinct from physics.

Traditional chemistry starts with the study of elementary particles, atoms, molecules, substances, metals, crystals and other aggregates of matter. in solid, liquid, and gas states, whether in isolation or combination. The interactions, reactions and transformations that are studied in chemistry are a result of interaction either between different chemical substances or between matter and energy.

A chemical reaction is a transformation of some substances into one or more different substances.

It can be symbolically depicted through a chemical equation. The number of atoms on the left and the right in the equation for a chemical transformation is most often equal. The nature of chemical reactions a substance may undergo and the energy changes that may accompany it are constrained by certain basic rules, known as chemical laws.

Energy and entropy considerations are invariably important in almost all chemical studies.

Chemical substances are classified in terms of their structure, phase as well as their chemical compositions. They can be analyzed using the tools of chemical analysis, e.g. spectroscopy and chromatography. Scientists engaged in chemical research are known as chemists. Most chemists specialize in one or more sub-disciplines. [8]

Basic Concepts in Chemistry

Atoms

Atoms are some of the basic building blocks of matter. Each atom is an element—an identifiable substance that cannot be further broken down into other identifiable substances.

There are just over 100 such elements, and each of them can combine with themselves and with other elements to create all the various molecules that exist in the universe. The poison gas chlorine and the explosive metal sodium, for instance, can combine at the atomic level to form sodium chloride, also known as salt.

For thousands of years atoms were thought to be the smallest thing possible. (The word "atom" comes from an ancient Greek word meaning "unbreakable.") However, experiments performed in the mid to late 19th century began to show the presence of small particles, electrons, in electric current. By the early 20th century, the electron was known to be a part of the atom that orbited a yet undefined atomic core. A few years later, in 1919, the proton was discovered and found to exist in the nuclei of all atoms.

The protons and neutrons inside an atomic nucleus are not fundamental particles. That is, they can be divided into still smaller pieces.

Protons and neutrons are known as hadrons, which is a class of particle made up of quarks. (Quarks are a fundamental particle.) There are two distinct types of hadrons, baryons and mesons, and both protons and neutrons are baryons, meaning they are both made up of a combination of three quarks. Besides being hadrons, protons and neutrons are also known as nucleons because of their place within the nucleus. Protons have a mass of around 1.6726×10^{-27} kg and neutrons have a nearly identical mass of 1.6929×10^{-27} kg. Both particles have a ½ spin.

The number of protons inside an atomic nucleus determines what element the atom is.

An element with only one proton, for instance, is hydrogen. An element with two is helium. One with three is lithium, and so on. No element (except for hydrogen) can exist with only protons in its nucleus. Atoms need neutrons to bond the protons together using the strong force. In general atoms (again except for hydrogen) have an equal number of protons and neutrons in their nuclei.

Atoms with an uneven number of protons and neutrons are called isotopes.

Isotopes have all the same chemical properties as their evenly balanced counterparts, but their nuclei are not usually as stable and are more willing to react with other elements. (Two deuterium atoms, hydrogen isotopes with one proton and one neutron in their nucleus rather than only one proton, will fuse much more readily than two regular hydrogen atoms.)

Nearly all of an atoms' mass is within its nucleus. Outside that there is a lot of empty space occupied only by a few, tiny electrons.

Electrons were once viewed as orbiting an atom like planets orbit the sun. We now know that this is wrong in several ways. For one, electrons do not really "orbit" in the sense we are used to. At the quantum level no particle is really a particle, but is actually both a particle and a wave simultaneously. Heisenberg's uncertainty principle looks at this odd truth about reality and says that you can never watch an electron orbit the nucleus as you would watch the Earth orbit the sun. Instead, you have to observe only one of the electron's physical characteristics at a time, either viewing it as a particle in a fixed position outside the nucleus or as a wave encircling the nucleus like a halo.

Additionally, planets orbiting their stars can orbit at any distance they want. In fact, every object in our solar system has an elliptical orbit, meaning that they all move in more oval rather than circular shapes, getting closer and farther from the sun at various points. Electrons cannot do this under any circumstances.

Atoms have what are known as electron shells, which are the levels that an electron is able to occupy.

Electrons cannot exist in between these shells; instead they jump from one to the next instantaneously. Each electron shell can hold a different number of atoms. When a shell fills up, additional electrons fill the outer shells. The outermost shell of any atom is called the valence shell, and it is the electrons in this shell that interact with the electrons of other atoms. The important thing about the valence shell is that each electron shell has a specific number of electrons that it can hold, and it wants to hold that many.

When atoms join together; their connecting valence electrons take up two valence shell spots, one on each atom.

This means that the fewer electrons an atom has in its valence shell, the likelier it is to interact with other atoms. Conversely, the more electrons it has, the less likely it is to interact.

Electrons can also momentarily jump from one electron shell to the next if they are hit with a burst of energy from a photon.

When photons hit atoms, the energy is briefly absorbed by the electrons, and this momentarily knocks them into higher "orbits." The particular "orbit" the electron is knocked into depends on the type of atom, and when the electron gives up its higher energy level it re-emits a photon at a slightly different wavelength than the one it absorbed, providing a characteristic signal of that atom and showing exactly what "orbit" the electron was knocked into.

This is the phenomenon responsible for spectral lines in light and is the reason we can tell what elements make up stars and planets just by looking at them.

Unlike protons and neutrons, electrons are a fundamental particle all on their own. They are known as leptons.

Electrons have a negative charge that is generally balanced out by the positive charge of their atom's protons.

Charged atoms, which have either gained or lost an electron for various reasons, are called ions.

Ions, like isotopes, have the same properties that the regular element does; they simply have different tendencies towards reacting with other atoms. Electrons have a mass of $9.1094 \times 10\text{-}31$ kg and a $-\frac{1}{2}$ spin.

Element

The concept of chemical element is related to that of chemical substance. A chemical element is specifically a substance which is composed of a single type of atom.

A chemical element is characterized by a particular number of protons in the nuclei of its atoms. This number is known as the atomic number of the element. For example, all atoms with 6 protons in their nuclei are atoms of the chemical element carbon, and all atoms with 92 protons in their nuclei are atoms of the element uranium.

Compound

A compound is a substance with a particular ratio of atoms of particular chemical elements which determines its composition, and a particular organization which determines chemical properties.

For example, water is a compound containing hydrogen and oxygen in the ratio of two to one, with the oxygen atom between the two hydrogen atoms, and an angle of $104.5°$ between them. Compounds are formed and interconverted by chemical reactions.

Substance

A chemical substance is a kind of matter with a definite composition and set of properties.

Strictly speaking, a mixture of compounds, elements or compounds and elements is not a chemical substance, but it may be called a chemical. Most of the substances we encounter in our daily life are some kind of mixture; for example: air, alloys, biomass, etc.

Nomenclature of substances is a critical part of the language of chemistry. Generally it refers to a system for naming chemical compounds.

Earlier in the history of chemistry substances were given names by their discoverer, which often led to some confusion and difficulty. However, today the IUPAC system of chemical nomenclature allows chemists to specify by name specific compounds amongst the vast variety of possible chemicals.

The standard nomenclature of chemical substances is set by the International Union of Pure and Applied Chemistry (IUPAC). There are well-defined systems in place for naming chemical species. Organic compounds are named according to the organic nomenclature system. Inorganic compounds are named according to the inorganic nomenclature system. In addition the Chemical Abstracts Service has devised a method to index chemical substance. In this scheme each chemical substance is identifiable by a number known as CAS registry number.

Molecule

Molecules are two or more atoms joined together through a chemical bond to form chemicals.

Molecules differ from atoms in that molecules can be further broken down into smaller pieces and into elements while atoms cannot. (This was actually the 18th century definition of an atom: a recognizable structure that could no longer be broken down into smaller bits.)

Atoms are joined together into molecules in two main ways: through covalent bonds and through ionic bonds.

Covalent bonds are the primary type of chemical bond that forms molecules. They occur when atoms with only partially filled valence electron shells, an atom's outermost electron shell, come together to share electrons. Hydrogen atoms, for instance, each have only one electron, while their valence shell is capable of holding two. When two hydrogen atoms come together each share the other's electron, using it to occupy its valence shell's free space forming the H2 molecule: hydrogen gas.

Not all covalent bond's are the same.

Different atoms have different levels of positive charge coming from in their nuclei, and although, under normal circumstances, the negative charge of the atom's electrons balances that out (keeping the atom electrically neutral) the chemical bonding process has a way of exploiting this situation. If we look at the H2 molecule again, everyday experience tells us that it has a strong tendency to seek out and bond with oxygen (O) molecules forming H20, or water. There are two main reasons for this. The first comes from the regular old covalent bonds that are already holding H2 together. If bonded to another atom, hydrogen gains the ability to form a new valence shell that can hold six electrons. Since oxygen is the only molecule to naturally have six electrons in its valence shell, it is the most eager to bond with hydrogen. However, oxygen also has 8 protons in its nucleus compared to the total of 2 in the H2 molecule. This means that as the atoms come closer and prepare to bond, the electrons from both atoms are pulled closer to the oxygen molecule and farther from the hydrogen. An atom's proclivity to pull electrons towards itself is called its electronegativity, and this process creates polar covalent bonds. Due to this connection, polar covalent bonds are the strongest molecular bond, which is why molecules like water are so prevalent in our solar system and, likely, throughout the galaxy.

One very interesting aspect of polar covalent bonds is the hydrogen bond.

When a hydrogen atom bonds with another electronegative atom, the newly created molecule develops an intense polar attraction to all other electronegative atoms. This attraction works almost like a magnet with one end of the molecule exhibiting a positive charge (due to the effects of the polar covalent bonds pulling all the electrons towards one end of the molecule) and the other end exhibiting a negative charge. This phenomenon is responsible for, among other things, the way water molecules stick to each other so readily. This is why you can fill a glass of water to a millimeter or so above the rim before it spills.

Hydrogen bonds are also responsible for how hydrophilic and hydrophobic molecules react to being mixed with water.

Hydrophilic molecules are molecules like NaCl (salt) which exhibit their own strong charge for reasons we will discuss in a moment. The charged salt molecules mix eagerly with the charged water molecules due to the extra pull of the hydrogen bond. Conversely, hydrophobic molecules such as oil will not mix with water because they are neutrally charged and do not like charged molecules. This is the reason you have to shake up an oil based salad dressing each time you use it. The oil and the water never truly mix, and given only a short amount of time they will separate.

A very different type of bond between atoms is called the ionic bond.

Ionic bonds only occur between ions, atoms that are either positively or negatively charged due to having an unequal number of protons and electrons. Ionic bonds always occur between metals and non-metals, such as the gas chlorine (Cl) and the alkaline metal sodium (Na). In their normal states, neither of these elements are ions, but when they approach each other, the sodium gives the chlorine one of its electrons forming Cl- and Na+ ions, which subsequently become attracted. Since no electrons are actually lost, the molecule still technically has a neutral charge; it is only the atoms that are charged.

In ionic bonds it is always the metal which gives its electron to the non-metal. Additionally, in a diluted or liquid form, molecules that are created like this will always conduct electricity. This is why salt water can make such a good conductor.

Ions and salts

An ion is a charged species, an atom or a molecule, that has lost or gained one or more electrons.

Positively charged cations (e.g. sodium cation Na+) and negatively charged anions (e.g. chloride Cl−) can form a crystalline lattice of neutral salts (e.g. sodium chloride NaCl). Examples of polyatomic ions that do not split up during acid-base reactions are hydroxide (OH−) and phosphate (PO43−).

Ions in the gaseous phase are often known as plasma.

Acidity and basicity

A substance can often be classified as an acid or a base. There are several different theories which explain acid-base behavior. The simplest is Arrhenius theory.

The Arrhenius theory states than an acid is a substance that produces hydronium ions when it is dissolved in water, and a base is one that produces hydroxide ions when dissolved in water. According to Brønsted–Lowry acid-base theory, acids are substances that donate a positive hydrogen ion to another substance in a chemical reaction; by extension, a base is the substance which receives that hydrogen ion.

A third common theory is Lewis acid-base theory, which is based on the formation of new chemical bonds.

Lewis theory explains that an acid is a substance which is capable of accepting a pair of electrons from another substance during the process of bond formation, while a base is a substance which can provide a pair of electrons to form a new bond. According to concept as per Lewis, the crucial things being exchanged are charges. There are several other ways in which a substance may be classified as an acid or a base, as is evident in the history of this concept

Acid strength is commonly measured by two methods. The most common is pH.

One measurement, based on the Arrhenius definition of acidity, is pH, which is a measurement of the hydronium ion concentration in a solution, as expressed on a negative logarithmic scale. Thus, solutions that have a low pH have a high hydronium ion concentration, and can be said to be more acidic. The other measurement, based on the Brønsted–Lowry definition, is the acid dissociation constant (Ka), which measure the relative ability of a substance to act as an acid under the Brønsted–Lowry definition of an acid. That is, substances with a higher Ka are more likely to donate hydrogen ions in chemical reactions than those with lower Ka values.

Phase

In addition to the specific chemical properties that distinguish chemical classifications, chemicals can exist in several phases.

For the most part, the chemical classifications are independent of these bulk phase classifications; however, some more exotic phases are incompatible with certain chemical properties. A phase is a set of states of a chemical system that have similar bulk structural properties, over a range of conditions, such as pressure or temperature.

Physical properties, such as density and refractive index tend to fall within values characteristic of the phase. The phase of matter is defined by the phase transition, which is when energy put into, or taken out of the system goes into rearranging the structure of the system, instead of changing the bulk conditions.

Phase can be continuous.

Sometimes the distinction between phases can be continuous instead of having a discrete boundary, here the matter is considered to be in a supercritical state. When three states meet based on the conditions, it is known as a triple point and since this is invariant, it is a convenient way to define a set of conditions.

The most familiar examples of phases are solids, liquids, and gases. Many substances exhibit multiple solid phases. For example, there are three phases of solid iron (alpha, gamma, and delta) that vary based on temperature and pressure. A principle difference between solid phases is the crystal structure, or arrangement, of the atoms. Another phase commonly encountered in the study of chemistry is the aqueous phase, which is the state of substances dissolved in aqueous solution (that is, in water).

Less familiar phases include plasmas, Bose-Einstein condensates and fermionic condensates and the paramagnetic and ferromagnetic phases of magnetic materials. While most familiar phases deal with three-dimensional systems, it is also possible to define analogs in two-dimensional systems, which has received attention for its relevance to systems in biology.

Redox

Redox is a concept related to the ability of atoms of various substances to lose or gain electrons.

Substances that have the ability to oxidize other substances are said to be oxidative and are known as oxidizing agents, oxidants or oxidizers. An oxidant removes electrons from another substance. Similarly, substances that have the ability to reduce other substances are said to be reductive and are known as reducing agents, reductants, or reducers.

A reductant transfers electrons to another substance, and is thus oxidized itself. And because it "donates" electrons it is also called an electron donor.

Oxidation and reduction properly refer to a change in oxidation number—the actual transfer of electrons may never occur. Thus, oxidation is better defined as an increase in oxidation number, and reduction as a decrease in oxidation number.

Bonding

Electron atomic and molecular orbitals

Atoms sticking together in molecules or crystals are said to be bonded with one another.

A chemical bond may be visualized as the multipole balance between the positive charges in the nuclei and the negative charges oscillating about them. More than simple attraction and repulsion, the energies and distributions characterize the availability of an electron to bond to another atom.

A chemical bond can be a covalent bond, an ionic bond, a hydrogen bond or just because of Van der Waals force.

Each of these kinds of bond is ascribed to some potential. These potentials create the interactions which hold atoms together in molecules or crystals. In many simple compounds, Valence Bond Theory, the Valence Shell Electron Pair Repulsion model (VSEPR), and the concept of oxidation number can be used to explain molecular structure and composition.

Reaction

During chemical reactions, bonds between atoms break and form, resulting in different substances with different properties.

In a blast furnace, iron oxide, a compound, reacts with carbon monoxide to form iron, one of the chemical elements, and carbon dioxide.

When a chemical substance is transformed as a result of its interaction with another or energy, a chemical reaction is said to have occurred. Chemical reaction is therefore a concept related to the 'reaction' of a substance when it comes in close contact with another, whether as a mixture or a solution; exposure to some form of energy, or, both. It results in some energy exchange between the constituents of the reaction as well with the system environment which may be designed vessels which are often laboratory glassware.

Chemical reactions can result in the formation or dissociation of molecules, that is, molecules breaking apart to form two or more smaller molecules, or rearrangement of atoms within or across molecules.

Chemical reactions usually involve the making or breaking of chemical bonds. Oxidation, reduction, dissociation, acid-base neutralization and molecular rearrangement are some of the commonly used kinds of chemical reactions.

A chemical reaction can be symbolically depicted through a chemical equation. While in a non-nuclear chemical reaction the number and kind of atoms on both sides of the equation are equal, for a nuclear reaction this holds true only for the nuclear particles viz. protons and neutrons.

The sequence of steps in which the reorganization of chemical bonds may be taking place in the course of a chemical reaction is called its mechanism.

A chemical reaction can be envisioned to take place in several steps, each of which may have a different speed. Many reaction intermediates with variable stability can thus be envisaged during a reaction. Reaction mechanisms are proposed to explain the kinetics and the relative product mix of a reaction. Many physical chemists specialize in exploring and proposing the mechanisms of various chemical reactions. Several empirical rules, like the Woodward-Hoffmann rules often come handy while proposing a mechanism for a chemical reaction.

Equilibrium

Although the concept of equilibrium is widely used across sciences, in the context of chemistry, it arises whenever a number of different states of the

chemical composition are possible.

For example, in a mixture of several chemical compounds that can react, or, when a substance can be present in more than one kind of phase.

A system of chemical substances at equilibrium even though having an unchanging composition is most often not static; molecules of the substances continue to react, thus creating a dynamic equilibrium. Thus the concept describes the state in which the parameters such as chemical composition remain unchanged over time. Chemicals present in biological systems are invariably not at equilibrium; but are far from equilibrium.

The Periodic Table

The periodic table contains the known chemical elements displayed in a special tabular arrangement based on their electron configurations, atomic numbers and recurring chemical properties.

The first semblance of a periodic table was by Antoine Lavoisier in 1789. He published a list or table of the 33 chemical elements known as of that time. He grouped the elements into earths, non-metals, gases and metals. The next century after that discovery saw several chemists looking for a better classification method and this gave rise to the periodic table as we have it today.

Structure of the Periodic Table

The standard periodic table as it is today is an 18 column by 7 rows table containing the main chemical elements. Beneath that is a smaller 15 column by 2 rows table. The periodic table can be broken down into 4 rectangular blocks: the P block is by the right, S block is left, D block is at the middle and the F block is underneath that. The elements in the blocks are based on which sub-shell the last electron resides.

The chemical elements on the table are arranged in order of increasing atomic number, which refers to the number of protons of the element. The periodic table can be used to study the chemical behavior of chemical elements, which makes it a very important tool widely used in chemistry.

The periodic table contains only chemical elements. Mixtures, compounds or small atomic particles of elements are not included. Each element on the table has a unique atomic number, which represents the number of protons contained in the element's nucleus.

A new period or row begins when an element has a new electron shell with a first electron. Columns or groups are based on the configuration of electrons of the atom. Elements that have an equal number of atoms in a specific sub-shell are listed under the same column. For example, selenium and oxygen both have 4 electrons in their outermost sub shell and so are listed under the P column. Elements with similar properties are listed in the same group although some elements in the same period can also share similar properties too. Since the elements grouped together have related properties, one can easily predict the property of an element if the properties of the surrounding elements are already known.

Rows are Periods

The rows of the periodic table are referred to as periods. Elements on a row have the same number of electron shells or atomic orbitals. Elements on the first row have just one atomic orbital, elements on the second row have 2, and so it goes until the elements on the seventh row that have 7 electron shells or atomic orbitals.

Columns are Groups

Columns from up to down in the table are called groups. The columns in the D, P and S blocks are called groups. Elements within a group have equal number of electrons in their outermost electron shell or orbital. The electrons on the outer shell are called valence electrons and there are the electrons that combine with other elements in a chemical reaction.

The Periodic table contains natural and synthesized elements

The elements up to californium are natural existing elements (94) while the rest were laboratory synthesized. Chemists are still working to produce elements beyond the present 118th element, ununoctium. 114 of the 118 elements on the table have been officially recognized by the International Union of Pure and Applied Chemistry (IUPAC). Elements listed on the table under 113, 115, 117 and 118 have been synthesized but are yet to officially recognized by the IUPAC and are only known by their systematic element names.

Chemistry and Energy

In the context of chemistry, energy is an attribute of a substance as a consequence of its atomic, molecular or aggregate structure. Since a chemical transformation is accompanied by a change in one or more of these kinds of structure, it is invariably accompanied by an increase or decrease of energy of the substances involved.

Some energy is transferred between the surroundings and the reactants of the reaction as heat or light; thus the products of a reaction may have more or less energy than the reactants.

Exergonic, Endergonic, Exothermic and Endothermic

A reaction is said to be exergonic if the final state is lower on the energy scale than the initial state; for endergonic reactions the situation is the reverse. A reaction is said to be exothermic if the reaction releases heat to the surroundings; for endothermic reactions, the reaction absorbs heat from the surroundings.

Chemical reactions are invariably not possible unless the reactants surmount an energy barrier known as the activation energy.

The speed of a chemical reaction (at given temperature T) is related to the activation energy E, by the Boltzmann's population factor $e - E / kT$ - that is the probability of molecule to have energy greater than than, or equal to E at the given temperature T. This exponential dependence of a reaction rate on temperature is known as the Arrhenius equation. The activation energy necessary for a chemical reaction can be in the form of heat, light, electricity or mechanical force as ultrasound.

Basic Physics

Kinetic and Mechanical Energy

The kinetic energy of an object is the energy it possesses due to its motion.

Kinetic energy is the work needed to accelerate a body of a given mass from rest to a stated velocity. Like all forms of energy, kinetic energy is measured in joules. Kinetic energy can be imparted to an object when an energy source is tapped to accelerate it. It can also happen when one object with kinetic energy slams into another object and kinetic energy from the first object is transferred to the second.

However it happens, imparting kinetic energy to an object causes it to accelerate. In this way movement is nothing more than an indication of the amount of kinetic energy an object has. An object will hold onto its kinetic energy until it is able to transfer it to something else, which allows it to slow down again.

As long as an object has the same level of kinetic energy, it will move at a consistent velocity forever. This is Newton's first law of motion.

The transfer of kinetic energy from one object to another can occur in many ways.

The transfer of kinetic energy can be as simple and mundane as a baseball flying through the air—interacting with all the various molecules of oxygen, carbon dioxide, nitrogen and all the other gasses that make up our atmosphere, and transferring its kinetic energy to them—speeding them up and slowing itself down in the process. Or it can be as chaotic as a speeding truck losing control on an icy road and slamming into a wall.

Different types of interactions between objects appear to be different but are in fact the same.

The interaction between the baseball and the air and between the truck and the wall are only superficially different. One appears more chaotic than the other only because of the differences in mass between a baseball and a truck and the differences in "negative energy" possessed by free-floating air molecules compared to a solid wall. At its most basic, however, the same events are taking place in both examples. Molecules both in the wall and the air scatter when the kinetic energy they receive causes them to move, and this causes both heat and sound to be produced.

Kinetic energy can be calculated with the formula KE=½mv² where m is the mass of the object in kilograms, and v is its velocity in meters/second.

Kinetic energy increases by the square of an objects velocity.

One important aspect of kinetic energy that makes it so potentially destructive is that the kinetic energy a moving object carries does not increase on pace with its velocity, but rather in relation to the square of its velocity. If you double an object's velocity, you will quadruple the amount of kinetic energy it possesses (22=4). If you quadruple the velocity, you increase the kinetic energy by sixteen times (42=16). This can lead to relatively small masses possessing very high kinetic energy levels when they are accelerated to only nominally high speeds. This is one reason why modern kinetic energy weapons (such as firearms) are able to cause large amounts of damage while being extremely compact.

Mechanical Energy

Mechanical energy is the ability of an object to do work.

When discussing energy it is important to take a moment to understand mechanical energy and how it relates to the objects it interacts with. Mechanical energy is not a separate type of energy in the way that potential energy and kinetic energy differ.

Mechanical energy is the potential energy available to an object added to all of the kinetic energy available to it, providing a total energy output.

For instance, in our description of potential energy there is the example of a pole-vaulter hanging in mid-air with her pole bent at a near right angle to the ground. The bend in the pole-vaulter's pole contains elastic potential energy, which will help her clear the bar. However, that is not the only source of energy the pole-vaulter is restricted to. For anyone who has ever seen a track and field competition, you know that pole-vaulters take long, running starts before planting their poles in the ground. This imparts kinetic energy to the runners body, and it is that kinetic energy plus the pole's elastic potential energy that are added together in mid-air to impart the total mechanical energy that drives the pole-vaulter high into the air and over the bar.

Potential Energy

There are two main types of potential energy: gravitational potential energy and elastic potential energy.

Potential energy is the potential an object has to act on other objects. As gravitational potential energy, the object is raised off the ground and is waiting for the force of gravity pulling at 9.8m/s^2, to grab hold of it and pull it towards the Earth.

This type of energy is very common in everyday life. It describes everything from a book falling off its shelf to a child tripping on a crack in the sidewalk. Because gravitational potential energy is so common, the equation describing it PEgrav=mass*g*height should not be hard to figure out since it contains only easily observable features of matter: an object's mass, the force of gravity (g), and the object's height off the ground when it started falling.

Note that the height does not have to be measured from the ground. Any point can be chosen—such as a table top or even a point in mid-air—provided that you are only concerned with the energy an object would have if it fell from the point it was currently at to the point you have chosen.

Gravitational Potential Energy Example

If we take the example of a 1kg weight positioned at a height of 1 meter above the surface of Earth (where the gravity is 9.8m/s^2—try this on Mars and you will get a different result), we end with the equation PEgrav=1*9.8*1, which equals 9.8 joules of gravitational potential energy. A 1g weight positioned at the same height would be PEgrav=.001*9.8*1 or .0098J of potential energy, while a 1kg weight positioned a kilometer up would equal PEgrav=1*9.8*1000 or 9800J of potential energy.
From this equation you may have picked up on the fact that the height an object is raised, is directly proportional to the amount of gravitational potential energy it has. Take a 1kg object and raise it to 5m, and you get 49J of potential energy. Double that to 10m, and you get 98J. Triple it to 15m and you will get 147J—three times the original 49J.

Elastic Potential Energy

Elastic potential energy occurs when an object is stretched or compressed out of its normal "resting" shape. The quantity of energy that will be released when it finally returns to rest is the quantity of elastic potential

energy it has while stretched or compressed.

A common example of elastic potential energy is when an archer draws back the string of his bow. The farther back the bowstring is pulled, the more it will stretch. The more it stretches the more potential energy it will have waiting to send into the arrow.

Elastic potential energy of an object can be determined using Hooke's law of elasticity. Hooke's law states that F=-kx where F is the force the material will exert as it returns to its resting state measured in Newtons, x is amount of displacement the material undergoes measured in meters, and k is the spring constant and is measured in Newtons/meter.

To determine the potential energy of an elastic or springy material you use the equation $PE = 1/2\ kx^2$. According to this equation, an object such as a spring with a spring constant of 5N/m that is stretched 3 meters past its resting point would have a potential energy of 22.5J. That is, ½*5*32 = 2.5*9 = 22.5J.

Remember that elastic potential energy affects much more than just what you would consider elastic or springy material such as rubber bands, bungee cords and springs. There is elastic potential energy in a pole-vaulter's pole at the point where she is in the air and hanging onto a pole that is bent nearly sideways. In the next instant her forward momentum will be boosted by the conversion of her pole's potential energy into kinetic energy, pushing her over the bar. Similarly, when a hockey player shoots the puck, he drags his stick along the ice as it moves forward, bending the shaft backwards slightly. This adds extra force to the puck as the stick snaps forward back into its normal resting position.

Energy: Work and Power

In the simplest terms, energy is the ability to do work.

Energy allows objects and people to affect the physical world and displace (or move) other objects or people.

Work in the physics sense is a very specific concept.

It is measured in joules, which are defined as being 1 Newton of force that displaces something by 1 meter. (J=Nm) As the mass of the object being displaced varies, the quantity of work in joules required to move it a meter will vary too.

To determine the quantity of work being done, you can use the equation W=F*d*cosΘ.

This defines work as the force applied, multiplied by the distance the object was displaced, multiplied by the cosine of Θ (Theta).

The force is measured in Newtons. Distance is measured in meters. The tricky part of this equation is determining the cosine of Θ. Θ represents the difference in angle between the vector (or direction) the force is acting in and the vector the displacement is occurring. That means that there are really only three possible values for Θ.

If the force is pushing or pulling in one direction, and the object being displaced is moving in that same direction, then there is no difference in angle between the vectors and Θ=0°. This is the sort of force you get when a child pulls her sled across a snowy field. The direction the child is pulling and the direction the sled is traveling are the same. Since cos0=1 the athe quantity of worketermined simply by multiplying the force and the displacement.

You should note that the angle of the vectors is determined by their relationship, and not to an ideal flat surface. That is, if the child is pulling her sled up a steep hill rather than across a field, the angle of Θ is still going to be 0° since the force she exerts on the sled and the sled itself are still traveling in the same direction.

The second possibility is when the force vector acts in the opposite direction of the object's displacement. This gives what is called "negative work" because the energy is working to hinder the object from moving rather than to help it. In this instance Θ=180° since the vector in which the force is acting and the vector in which the object is moving are opposite. This force is most commonly observed when dealing with friction. It is the reason that hockey pucks and soccer balls will not travel forever; the force of friction exerted by the ice and by the grass is acting in the opposite direction.

The final difference in vectors is when the force being exerted on an object is at a right angle to its displacement. In this case Θ=90°. You can picture this as a waitress carrying a tray of drinks over to your table, and it provides for some odd conclusions. Since the force we are talking about is the force the waitress is using to hold the tray vertically, but the displacement vector of the tray is horizontally across the room, we find that the force the waitress exerts does no work at all. It is not responsible for moving the tray horizontally towards your table.
This is represented mathematically with the fact that the cos90=0,

meaning that the original equation W=F*d*cosϴ would be W=F*d*0. Without adding any other information in, it is already obvious that work is going to equal zero joules.

A different way to imagine this is to think of cargo in the back of a truck.

It took work to load the cargo up onto the truck from the ground (the force vector and the displacement vector were both pointing in the same direction), but once the cargo was loaded, no additional work was required to keep it there. The truck could drive from one end of the country to the other, but zero joules of work would be exerted keeping the cargo in place in the back of the truck.

When you add a unit of time to your calculations of work, you get a new classification: power.

Power is the rate at which work is done. The equation that measures power is power=work/time. In this equation work is measured in joules, time is measured in seconds and power is measured in watts. Since, as we noted above, one joule is the same as one Newton multiplied by one meter, this equation can also be written as power=(force*displacement)/time where force is measured in Newtons and displacement is measured in meters. However, this opens up further possibilities. Since the math does not care whether we first multiply force with displacement before dividing the whole thing by time, or whether we divide displacement by time and then multiply the answer by force, we find the equation can also be written as power=force(displacement/time).

Given that displacement is measured in meters and the time in seconds, what we are really saying here is that power equals the amount of force applied to an object multiplied by that object's velocity (m/s).

Thus we get two equations describing power: power=work/time and power=force*velocity.

By definition, power has an inverse relationship with time; the less time that it takes for the work to be done, the more power is being applied. Power also has a direct relationship with force and velocity. Increase either the quantity of force being applied to an object, or the speed at which it is traveling, and you have increased the power.

Defining Force and Newton's Three Laws

In physics force is the term given to anything that has the power to act on an object, causing its displacement in one direction or another.

Forces are a somewhat abstract concept, and therefore it took thousands of years to accurately identify and describe them. It was not until the 17th century when a man named Isaac Newton began to accurately describe the basic physical forces and show how they acted on matter.

Force is measured using the unit Newton (N). One Newton can be defined with the formula $1N = 1kg(1m/s^2)$. In other words, if you accelerate a kilogram of matter by one meter per second per second, you have exerted one Newton of force on it.

Newton developed three laws to explain the interactions of matter he observed. The first is often known as the "Law of Inertia."

It states that an object at rest will stay at rest, and an object in motion will stay in motion, unless a force acts upon it to change its state. This means that if you fire a spaceship out into the vacuum of space, and keep it clear from planets and stars that will apply force to it, the ship will keep going at the same speed forever.

This tendency to stay moving or stay at rest is known as inertia. Inertia is directly related to an object's mass; the more mass an object has, the more inertia it will have and the harder it will be to speed it up or slow it down. This is implied by the equation defining one Newton of force, but it is also obvious in everyday life. You have to exert more force to push a box of books across the floor than you would to push a box of clothes the same size. The box of books has more mass, so it has more inertia. Similarly, a baseball player can easily catch and stop a baseball thrown at over 100km/hr. If you were to ask that same player to stop a truck traveling at 100km/hr, you would get much less pleasant results.

One important thing to remember about force is that it is a vector quantity, meaning that it points in a specific direction.

Set a one kilogram object down on a table and you will have the force of gravity pulling it down at one Newton, and the force of all the atoms in the table pushing it up at one Newton. This is said to be a state of equilibrium, and it causes no change to the object's velocity. However, if the table had been poorly built and was only capable of pushing up at .75 Newtons, the object would pull through, snapping the table at its weakest points, and fall until it found something that was capable of applying the needed force to hold it up against gravity.

As such, an object can only be at rest if it has no forces acting on it, or if it has equal and opposite forces acting on it keeping it at equilibrium. If an unopposed force acts on an object, it will move.

Newton's second law deals with what happens when you have the sort of unbalanced forces that we just described.

It explains the movement of objects through the equation F=ma, where F is the force in Newtons, m is the object's mass in kilograms, and a is the object's acceleration in meters per second per second (m/s2).
Just like with Newton's first law, this equation shows that mass is a huge player when it comes to using a force to move objects. The larger the mass, the more force you will need to accelerate or decelerate it to the same velocity.

Newton's third law states simply that for every action there is an equal and opposite reaction.

This means that if I pound my hand down on my desk right now, my desk will also be hitting up at my hand with the exact same force. This may sound strange, but it is the reason that pounding your hand on your desk can damage your desk and hurt your hand at the same time. It is also the reason that baseball bats can snap while imparting force onto the ball, and why a moving car hitting stationary wall will damage both.

Force: Friction

Friction is the force that resists the motion of objects in relation to other objects.

When two surfaces move relative to each other, the force of friction is what slows them down. Friction applies to all matter, whether it is a book sliding down a slanting shelf, a soccer ball rolling on the ground or a baseball flying though the air. Friction is a constant opposing force that keeps things from traveling forever.

Several laws describe how friction works.

Amontons' first law of friction says that, "The force of friction is directly proportional to the applied load." His second law of friction says that, "The force of friction is independent of the apparent area of contact." Similarly,

Coulomb's law of friction states that, "Kinetic friction is independent of the sliding velocity."

The two main types of Friction are static friction and kinetic friction.

Static friction is what you get when one stationary object is stacked on top of another stationary object, such as a book resting on a table. The static friction between the book and the table determines how much sticking power there is between them, and at what angle you would have to tilt the table before the force of gravity overpowers the force of friction and starts the book sliding.

To figure out the maximum amount of static friction possible before the book starts sliding, you use the formula $f_s = \mu_s F_n$ where f_s is the total amount of static friction, μ_s (pronounced "mu") is the coefficient of static friction and F_n is the "normal force," the force being exerted perpendicularly through the surface into the object resting on it, keeping the object from breaking through the surface.

Another way to examine static friction is to calculate the angle the table will have to reach before the book will start sliding.

This is also known as the angle of repose, and it can be calculated using the formula $\tan\theta = \mu_s$ where θ (pronounced "theta") is the angle of repose and μ_s is the coefficient of static friction.

Aside from determining the angels that books will slide off tables, calculating static friction allows tire manufacturers to determine how "grippy" their treads are. If there were no friction, the wheel would not be a functional tool because it would not push itself against the road while moving. The higher the coefficient of friction between the tire and the road, the more grip the tire has.

Kinetic friction is sort of the inverse of static friction.

It is the force that causes moving objects to slow down. Kinetic friction applies to two surfaces moving in respect to one another such as the bottom of a snowboard and the snowy ground. It can be calculated using the same basic formula used to calculate static friction: $f_k = \mu_k F_n$ with the only differences being the sub-k marks replacing the sub-s marks of the previous equation, signifying kinetic friction.

As kinetic friction slows an object, the object's kinetic energy is transformed into heat.

Fundamental Forces: Electromagnetism

Electromagnetism is one of the four fundamental forces. It is far more common than gravity, but only if you know where to look.

Electromagnetism is responsible for nearly all interactions in which gravity plays no part. It is what holds negatively charged electrons in orbit around the positively charged protons in the nucleus of an atom. It is also the force that joins atoms to each other to create molecules.

It is also electromagnetism that is responsible for the fact that matter—which is made up of atoms and at the subatomic level is mostly empty space—feels solid.

When you sit down in your chair, it is the electromagnetic attraction between the chair's atoms and between your body's atoms that keep you from falling through the chair and, conversely, that keep the chair from passing through you.

Electromagnetic force acts through a field.

This type of field can occur as a result of positively or negatively charged atoms (ions), atoms which have either more or fewer electrons than protons causing their overall charge to be unbalanced. Magnetic fields can also be created by applying electric current to conductive material (such as wire) with a conductive core (such as a nail).

Electric current is nothing more than a steady flow of electrons, and by turning on the current you send electrons through the core.

This aligns all the atoms in the metal so that they are parallel, and this creates a magnetic field. When you turn the electric current off, the electrons stop flowing, and the atoms, no longer forced by the current to line up, cease to be magnetic.

All electromagnetic fields have a positive and a negative pole.

Even the Earth's magnetic field, which is caused by the convective forces in the planet's core, sends electrons out of its negative pole (in the geographic North Pole) and reaccepts them at its positive pole (in the geographic South Pole in Antarctica). The Earth's magnetic field, like all magnetic fields, is able to effect charged particles.

Magnetic fields move in one direction around a magnet.

This direction is always the same in relation to the flow of current from the negative to the positive poles, and it is easy to test the direction of the field using the "right hand rule." Close your fist and make a "thumbs up" sign with your right hand. The positive pole is represented by the tip of your thumb, the negative by the other end of your hand, and the direction of the magnetic field by where your closed fingers are. Thus, if you point your thumb at yourself, your magnet has current coming out its negative pole pointed towards you and looping back around to the positive pole pointed away from you, and the field is pointed counter-clockwise, which here is to your left.

The effects of a magnetic field do not go on forever but follow the inverse square law.

The farther you move from a magnetic field, the less its force will affect you. By moving x times away from a magnetic field, you feel $1/x2$ times less magnetism.

Closely related to the electromagnetic field is electromagnetic radiation.

This radiation can take many forms, the most familiar of which being light, radio waves that carry radio and broadcast television, microwaves that cook our food, x-rays that can image the insides or our bodies, and gamma rays that come down from space and would have killed us all long ago if it were not for the Earth's magnetic field interacting with them.

Electromagnetic radiation is created, according to James Clerk Maxwell, by the oscillations of electromagnetic fields, which create electromagnetic waves.

The wave's frequency (or how energetic it is) determines what part of the electromagnetic spectrum it occupies—whether it is a gamma ray, a blue light or a radio signal. Electromagnetic radiation is the same thing as light, with what we are used to as visible light being a range of specific frequencies within the electromagnetic spectrum, so all electromagnetic radiation moves at the speed of light.

At the quantum level, the electromagnetic force has a transfer particle moving back and forth between charged atoms, attracting and repelling them. The electromagnetic transfer particle is the photon.

Fundamental Forces: Gravity

Gravity may be the most commonly, consciously experienced force.

We can see its effects everyday when books fall off shelves, when stray baseballs arc downwards and crash through windows and when Australians time and again fail to fall off the bottom of the world and out into space. Gravity is also largely responsible for the structure of the universe. Without it, stars would not ignite and begin fusion reactions, planets would not condense out of dust and metal and most matter would have no attraction to other matter in any way. Without gravity, life would not exist.

It may seem strange to learn that gravity is the weakest of all forces given that it holds the entire galaxy together.

Still, even with the gravitational mass of the entire planet pulling on an object such as a ball—causing it to sit motionless on the floor rather than float aimlessly off into space—a toddler could easily pick it up and run off with it, and there would be nothing the planet could do about it. Match that with the force an electromagnet exerts on metal; there is no comparison.

The idea of gravity as a force was first formulated by Isaac Newton in the late 17th century.

Newton's ideas were further elaborated on in the early 20th century by Albert Einstein, who described gravity as the effect of mass warping the fabric of space-time. This process is often portrayed as a large ball creating a divot in a flat sheet of space-time. The divot curves space-time and can catch objects that would otherwise be traveling in straight lines and redirect or even capture them.

On Earth gravity pulls objects towards the center of the planet at 9.8 m/s^2.

The squared rate of time shows that gravity is by its nature a force causing acceleration. Every second, the force of gravity increases the speed of an object by an additional 9.8 m/s, provided nothing able to resist the force gets in its way.

In Einstein's view of the universe, gravity moved in waves, which traveled through space at the speed of light.

As a result, he demonstrated that the force of gravity would take time to reach the object it was acting on. If, for instance, the sun were to vanish suddenly from the solar system, it would take eight minutes for the Earth to go flying off into space—the same amount of time it would take for us to stop seeing the sun's light.

Another way to view gravity is through a series of transfer particles that interact with matter and draw it closer together.

Transfer particles come into play in quantum mechanics, and they replace gravity waves as the method of spreading the force through the universe. (Actually, replace is not the right word, as quantum mechanics shows that particles and waves are really the same thing, simply looked at from different perspectives.) In quantum mechanics gravity's transfer particle is called a graviton, and it moves at the speed of light.

The farther you move from a gravitational mass, the less its force will affect you.

The drop in the gravitational force is governed by what is known as the inverse square law, which says that the attraction of any object drops in relation to the square of the distance you move from it. If you are floating over the surface of the planet and then move x times away from it, you will feel $1/x^2$ times less gravity. So if you move 10 times farther away from where you were, you will feel $1/100$ the force gravity.

Fundamental Forces: Strong and Weak Nuclear Forces

The strong and weak nuclear forces are fundamental forces, but they were discovered much later than electromagnetism and gravity primarily because they only interact with matter at a subatomic level.

Strong nuclear force is the strongest of the four fundamental forces.

Strong nuclear force is 100 times stronger than the next strongest force, electromagnetism, and 1036 times the strength of the weakest force, gravity. That said, for the thousands of years that people have been studying physics, it never occurred to any one to even look for the strong force. That is because, despite the strong force's strength, it has such a limited range that it only interacts with matter across the distance of an atom's nucleus. In fact, its range is only about 10-15 meters, so small that the nuclei of the largest atoms—those filled with the highest number of protons and neutrons—are only just barely small enough for the strong force to keep working, making the nuclei of those atoms unstable.

The strong force was not discovered until the 1930s when scientists discovered the neutron.

Until that time atomic nuclei were thought to consist of a collection of protons and electrons grouped together in such a way that kept them mutually attracted. With the discovery of the neutron, however, a new force was needed to hold positively charged protons together with uncharged neutrons.

Strong Nuclear force interacts with Quarks.

The strong force actually does not interact directly with the protons and neutrons but with the fundamental particle that makes up protons and neutrons, quarks. Quarks come in three different color groupings: red, green and blue. (Quarks are not actually these colors; red, green and blue are just familiar names given to bits of matter that are utterly outside our experience as humans, to make them easier to comprehend.) The different colors of quarks combine to create protons and neutrons. Within each proton and neutron, the strong force holds the quarks together. That, in turn, bleeds out into the rest of the nucleus in a residual effect, holding the protons and neutrons together as well.

Like the other fundamental forces, the strong force is mediated at the quantum level using a transfer particle known as a gluon. However, unlike the transfer particles for gravity and electromagnetism (gravitons and photons, respectively), gluons have mass. It is the gluon's mass that limits the area where it can spread the strong force to only within the nucleus.

Weak nuclear force causes a type of radioactive decay.

The other fundamental force operating inside the nucleus is the weak force. The weak force causes a specific type of radioactive decay called beta decay, so named because it causes the decaying atom to emit a beta particle, which can be either an electron or a positron (a form of anti-mater also known as an anti-electron), as a byproduct of changing into a different element.

Several things happen at once during beta decay, and we should look at each one individually. We saw while looking at the strong force that an atom's protons and neutrons are made up of smaller, fundamental particles called quarks, and it is the quarks that actually interact with the strong force. As it turns out, quarks are the only particle that interacts with all four fundamental forces, which means that inside the nucleus they are interacting with the weak force as well.

Besides three different colors: red, blue and green, Quarks can be divided into six different flavors: up, down, charm, strange, top and bottom.

Before we get to how the weak force interacts with quarks, there is something else you should know about them. We mentioned above that quarks come in three different colors: red, blue and green. However, they also can be divided into six different flavors: up, down, charm, strange, top and bottom. (This makes 18 different possible combinations of quark, each with a color and a flavor.) Of these flavors only up and down quarks are stable enough to form protons and neutrons.

What the weak force does is switch up quarks to down quarks and down quarks to up quarks.

This is actually the only thing that the weak force does, but it has several effects. First since quarks join to produce protons and neutrons (two up quarks and one down quark make a proton, while two down and one up quark make a neutron), the sudden change of one type of quark to another changes that combination. β− decay is beta decay where change of quarks causes a neutron to become a proton. This also causes the atom to emit an electron and a electron antineutrino. β + decay is the opposite, where a proton changes to a neutron and the atom emits a positron and an electron neutrino.

In both cases the decaying atom changes into a different kind of atom. In general, beta decay takes place in unstable isotopes (atoms that have a different number of protons and neutrons) and stabilizes the nucleus by equalizing the ratio of these particles. For instance, beta decay will turn the unstable plutonium 15 into far more stable strontium 16.

Quantum Mechanics

Quantum mechanics is the study of quanta, the most basic individual unit of any substance.

Quantum mechanics first began as a discipline within physics in 1900 when Max Planck determined that energy radiated as heat could not just radiate at any temperature, but that it could only rise and fall—and thus be emitted or absorbed—at certain, set levels. (Think of it as the difference between stairs and ramps. Stairs have set spaces where you can stand and set spaces where you cannot. Planck said that raising energy levels such as temperature was akin to climbing a set of stairs one step at a time.)

Radiation that produces heat (and thus all electromagnetic radiation, including visible light) is made up of tiny little particles, which Planck named quanta from the Latin work "quantus," which means "how much."

Planck developed an equation to describe this situation, E=hv in which v stood for the already well known frequencies of electromagnetic spectrum (and which in 1900 was thought of as only acting like a wave), h stood for a number called the Planck constant that equaled 6.63×10−34 J s ("J s" is for Joule seconds), and E was the energy level for quanta of that frequency.

In 1905 Albert Einstein used Planck's work to define the photon, which is one quantum of electromagnetic radiation.

Photons are generally thought of as light, but only some energies of photons are visible. Photons can have any energy that corresponds to electromagnetic frequency, but instead of being a continuous wave, they are thought of as individual particles.

Waves and particles are the same thing look at in different ways.

The discovery of the particle aspect of a wave lead to a realization that waves and particles were actually the same thing, looked at in different ways. This idea, called wave-particle duality, accounted for the centuries long debate between physicists over whether light was a wave or a particle, with each side producing compelling evidence to prove its thesis. As it turned out light—like everything in the universe—was both. This relationship was demonstrated by Louis de Broglie who developed the equation p=h/λ showing that the Planck constant (h) divided by a particle's wavelength (λ, pronounced lambda) would equal its momentum (p). Since all particles are moving and have momentum, all particles have wavelengths.

One of the most important aspects of wave-particle duality comes from studying atoms.

The orbits of electrons around the atomic nuclei had at one time been thought to mimic the orbits of planets around the sun. Now, however, two important factors came into play to change that view. The first was the realization that electrons could only orbit at certain distances from the nucleus. When changing from one electron shell to the next, an electron would not take a gradual trajectory to its new home in the way a spaceship from Earth to Mars might. The electron would simply vanish from one shell and appear instantaneously at the next. In essence, electrons could also only display certain quanta of energy. They could have one energy level or another, but they could not exist in between.

The second important thing that quantum mechanics showed physicists is that "orbit" does not describe electrons and is only symbolic.

Since all particles are also waves, an electron could not simply be in one place at one time, but had to exist as across a range of areas as a frequency which described its momentum.

The Heisenberg uncertainty principle states you can measure the position of an electron or the velocity, but not both at once.

This seemingly nonsensical idea was explained mathematically though the Heisenberg uncertainty principle, which stated that it was possible to measure the exact position of a particle, and it was possible to measure the exact velocity of a particle, but you could not know both factors at once. In other words, measuring one would make it impossible to measure the other. This was an unavoidable fact of reality given de Broglie's equation; if you were moving you were spread out like a wave.

No particles in the universe can be said to have definite positions in space.

A strange side effect of this was it meant that no particles in the universe could be said to have definite positions in space. Instead, everything had a likely position given its velocity. Matter could not be said to exist at certain points in space, it could merely have certain probabilities of existing at those points.

Gravity is still a problem.

The 21st century understanding of gravity comes from Einstein's work on Special and General Relativity. The various predictions made by Einstein's theories have been proven correct experimentally on numerous occasions, and evidently his ideas accurately explain reality. However, they do not mix with quantum mechanics.

Physics has three zones which do not mix - relativity, quantum mechanics and Newtonian.

It is possible to look at physics and think of there as being three distinct zones: relativity, which describes the very big and the very fast; quantum mechanics, which describes the very small; and Newtonian physics, which describes everything in between.

But Newtonian physics easily unifies with quantum theory since the chaos and weirdness at the individual wave-particle level smooths out as you add more and more particles together, which is what we see when we look at the macro world in which we live. (That is, when you look at an object in front of you, you see it existing in a definite point in space because so many particles make it up the probability that they will all end suddenly existing elsewhere—the way individual particles can—drops to nearly zero.) Additionally, three of the four fundamental forces, electromagnetism, the strong force and the weak force, can all be explained through quantum mechanics using their three transfer particles; photons, gluons and bosons. They have been unified. However, the use of a gravity transfer particle, the graviton, in models has been less successful at bringing the experimentally accurate predictions of relativity in line with the functioning of reality at the quantum level.

States of Matter

Matter on Earth can exist in three main states or phases: solid, liquid and gas. There is also a fourth phase, plasma, that occurs when matter is superheated.

The primary difference between the different phases of matter is the behavior of molecules relative to the temperature the matter is exposed to. The lower the temperature, the closer together and more locked together the molecules are. The higher the temperature, the farther apart the molecules are, and the more they move relative to one another.

Solid

Solid matter exists in a state where its molecules are locked together in a rigid structure preventing them from moving and, as a result, solid matter is held together in a specific shape.

There are two primary types of solids, each defined by the structures in which their molecules are held. When the molecules in solid matter maintain a uniform organization they form a polycrystalline structure. This is how molecules in metal, ice and salt are organized. Polycrystalline structures are generally a result of the molecules' ionic properties. Water molecules, for instance, are formed in such a way that there are distinct ends, one with two hydrogen atoms and one with a single oxygen atom. The structure of the atoms within a water molecule means these ends are charged, giving it what amount to poles and causing water molecules to join together only in specific patterns. Under a microscope polycrystalline solids are generally described as resembling lattice work or a chain link fence, with the same pattern of molecules from one end to the other.

When molecule's electromagnetic properties do not incline them to form into particular structures, they glob together in whatever patterns they can. This produces amorphous solids, most notably foams, glass and many types of plastic. Amorphous solids have no regular pattern throughout their structure and, as a result, are poor conductors of heat and electricity.

Liquid

When solids are heated past a certain point, the electromagnetic bonds holding their molecules together loosen, and the molecules are able to move more freely.

While the temperatures required for this to happen can vary widely, the particular physical qualities of a liquid are always the same. Liquids are considered to be fluids, which differ from solids primarily in their ability to take the shape of any container they are held in. This is the result of a less intense electromagnetic connection between the molecules than there is in solids; however, there is still enough of a that liquids still want to stay all in the same place. This is why liquids still maintain a low density that is nearly identical to their densities in solid form, and why they will maintain a constant volume rather than just drift off the way gasses do. Liquids also have a property known as viscosity, which describes their willingness to flow over and away from themselves. Liquids such as water and honey have a constant viscosity and are known as Newtonian fluids. Non-Newtonian fluids, such as a goopy mixture of water and cornstarch can change their viscosities.

Gas

The third state of matter that is commonly found on Earth is gas. Gasses are formed when matter is heated beyond its liquid state so that the electromagnetic bonds holding its molecules together are severed almost completely.

Gasses are also considered fluids and like liquids have no definite shape. But unlike liquids they also lack a definite volume and have an extremely low density compared to their solid forms.

Since gasses lack both a shape and a volume, they will expand to fill any container they are placed in. Left unbounded they will expand forever. Conversely, gasses are perfectly happy to compress together in an enclosed space. (However, the more molecules of a gas that are enclosed in a space together, the higher the gas's pressure—the force exerted by the molecules on the container's surface—will be.) One interesting thing about this expansion and compression is that it will always be homogeneous, meaning that as a gas expands to fill a container, there will never be pockets of a higher density of molecules in some areas with a lower density of molecules in others. The molecules will expand to fill the container equally.

Plasma

Plasma is the next step up from a gas; it is when a gas's molecules become super heated to the point where the molecular bonds themselves break down and the atoms begin shedding their electrons.

Although plasma is rarely found on Earth, it is the most common state of matter throughout the universe. (It is the primary state of matter in stars, for instance.) Plasma has some unique characteristics, not the least of which is that it is ionized, or electrically charged. In many ways plasma acts like a gas. It lacks any definite shape or volume, and it will homogeneously fill any container. However, it can also be manipulated by electromagnetic fields, which alters its shape or contains it. Plasma is a super-heated, magnetically charged gas.

Practice Test 1

Part 1 - Academic Aptitude

Verbal Sub-test – Vocabulary
Questions: 30
Time: 30 Minutes

Mathematics Sub-test
Questions: 30
Time: 30 Minutes

Nonverbal Sub-test
Questions: 30
Time: 30 Minutes

Part II – Spelling
Questions: 30
Time: 30 Minutes

Part III – Reading Comprehension
Questions: 35
Time: 35 Minutes

Part VI – Basic Science
Questions: 60
Time: 60 minutes

The practice test portion presents questions that are representative of the type of question you should expect to find on the PSB. However, they are not intended to match exactly what is on the PSB. Don't worry though! If you can answer these questions, you will have not trouble with the PSB.

For the best results, take this Practice Test as if it were the real exam. Set aside time when you will not be disturbed, and a location that is quiet and free of distractions. Read the instructions carefully, read each question carefully, and answer to the best of your ability.

Use the bubble answer sheets provided. When you have completed the Practice Test, check your answer against the Answer Key and read the explanation provided.

Answer Sheet – Part 1 – Vocabulary Sub-test

1. Ⓐ Ⓑ Ⓒ Ⓓ   11. Ⓐ Ⓑ Ⓒ Ⓓ   21. Ⓐ Ⓑ Ⓒ Ⓓ

2. Ⓐ Ⓑ Ⓒ Ⓓ   12. Ⓐ Ⓑ Ⓒ Ⓓ   22. Ⓐ Ⓑ Ⓒ Ⓓ

3. Ⓐ Ⓑ Ⓒ Ⓓ   13. Ⓐ Ⓑ Ⓒ Ⓓ   23. Ⓐ Ⓑ Ⓒ Ⓓ

4. Ⓐ Ⓑ Ⓒ Ⓓ   14. Ⓐ Ⓑ Ⓒ Ⓓ   24. Ⓐ Ⓑ Ⓒ Ⓓ

5. Ⓐ Ⓑ Ⓒ Ⓓ   15. Ⓐ Ⓑ Ⓒ Ⓓ   25. Ⓐ Ⓑ Ⓒ Ⓓ

6. Ⓐ Ⓑ Ⓒ Ⓓ   16. Ⓐ Ⓑ Ⓒ Ⓓ   26. Ⓐ Ⓑ Ⓒ Ⓓ

7. Ⓐ Ⓑ Ⓒ Ⓓ   17. Ⓐ Ⓑ Ⓒ Ⓓ   27. Ⓐ Ⓑ Ⓒ Ⓓ

8. Ⓐ Ⓑ Ⓒ Ⓓ   18. Ⓐ Ⓑ Ⓒ Ⓓ   28. Ⓐ Ⓑ Ⓒ Ⓓ

9. Ⓐ Ⓑ Ⓒ Ⓓ   19. Ⓐ Ⓑ Ⓒ Ⓓ   29. Ⓐ Ⓑ Ⓒ Ⓓ

10. Ⓐ Ⓑ Ⓒ Ⓓ   20. Ⓐ Ⓑ Ⓒ Ⓓ   30. Ⓐ Ⓑ Ⓒ Ⓓ

Answer Sheet – Part I – Mathematics Sub-test

1. (A) (B) (C) (D)　　11. (A) (B) (C) (D)　　21. (A) (B) (C) (D)

2. (A) (B) (C) (D)　　12. (A) (B) (C) (D)　　22. (A) (B) (C) (D)

3. (A) (B) (C) (D)　　13. (A) (B) (C) (D)　　23. (A) (B) (C) (D)

4. (A) (B) (C) (D)　　14. (A) (B) (C) (D)　　24. (A) (B) (C) (D)

5. (A) (B) (C) (D)　　15. (A) (B) (C) (D)　　25. (A) (B) (C) (D)

6. (A) (B) (C) (D)　　16. (A) (B) (C) (D)　　26. (A) (B) (C) (D)

7. (A) (B) (C) (D)　　17. (A) (B) (C) (D)　　27. (A) (B) (C) (D)

8. (A) (B) (C) (D)　　18. (A) (B) (C) (D)　　28. (A) (B) (C) (D)

9. (A) (B) (C) (D)　　19. (A) (B) (C) (D)　　29. (A) (B) (C) (D)

10. (A) (B) (C) (D)　　20. (A) (B) (C) (D)　　30. (A) (B) (C) (D)

Answer Sheet – Part I – Nonverbal Sub-test

1. Ⓐ Ⓑ Ⓒ Ⓓ   11. Ⓐ Ⓑ Ⓒ Ⓓ   21. Ⓐ Ⓑ Ⓒ Ⓓ

2. Ⓐ Ⓑ Ⓒ Ⓓ   12. Ⓐ Ⓑ Ⓒ Ⓓ   22. Ⓐ Ⓑ Ⓒ Ⓓ

3. Ⓐ Ⓑ Ⓒ Ⓓ   13. Ⓐ Ⓑ Ⓒ Ⓓ   23. Ⓐ Ⓑ Ⓒ Ⓓ

4. Ⓐ Ⓑ Ⓒ Ⓓ   14. Ⓐ Ⓑ Ⓒ Ⓓ   24. Ⓐ Ⓑ Ⓒ Ⓓ

5. Ⓐ Ⓑ Ⓒ Ⓓ   15. Ⓐ Ⓑ Ⓒ Ⓓ   25. Ⓐ Ⓑ Ⓒ Ⓓ

6. Ⓐ Ⓑ Ⓒ Ⓓ   16. Ⓐ Ⓑ Ⓒ Ⓓ   26. Ⓐ Ⓑ Ⓒ Ⓓ

7. Ⓐ Ⓑ Ⓒ Ⓓ   17. Ⓐ Ⓑ Ⓒ Ⓓ   27. Ⓐ Ⓑ Ⓒ Ⓓ

8. Ⓐ Ⓑ Ⓒ Ⓓ   18. Ⓐ Ⓑ Ⓒ Ⓓ   28. Ⓐ Ⓑ Ⓒ Ⓓ

9. Ⓐ Ⓑ Ⓒ Ⓓ   19. Ⓐ Ⓑ Ⓒ Ⓓ   29. Ⓐ Ⓑ Ⓒ Ⓓ

10. Ⓐ Ⓑ Ⓒ Ⓓ   20. Ⓐ Ⓑ Ⓒ Ⓓ   30. Ⓐ Ⓑ Ⓒ Ⓓ

Answer Sheet - Part II – Spelling

1. Ⓐ Ⓑ Ⓒ Ⓓ   11. Ⓐ Ⓑ Ⓒ Ⓓ   21. Ⓐ Ⓑ Ⓒ Ⓓ

2. Ⓐ Ⓑ Ⓒ Ⓓ   12. Ⓐ Ⓑ Ⓒ Ⓓ   22. Ⓐ Ⓑ Ⓒ Ⓓ

3. Ⓐ Ⓑ Ⓒ Ⓓ   13. Ⓐ Ⓑ Ⓒ Ⓓ   23. Ⓐ Ⓑ Ⓒ Ⓓ

4. Ⓐ Ⓑ Ⓒ Ⓓ   14. Ⓐ Ⓑ Ⓒ Ⓓ   24. Ⓐ Ⓑ Ⓒ Ⓓ

5. Ⓐ Ⓑ Ⓒ Ⓓ   15. Ⓐ Ⓑ Ⓒ Ⓓ   25. Ⓐ Ⓑ Ⓒ Ⓓ

6. Ⓐ Ⓑ Ⓒ Ⓓ   16. Ⓐ Ⓑ Ⓒ Ⓓ   26. Ⓐ Ⓑ Ⓒ Ⓓ

7. Ⓐ Ⓑ Ⓒ Ⓓ   17. Ⓐ Ⓑ Ⓒ Ⓓ   27. Ⓐ Ⓑ Ⓒ Ⓓ

8. Ⓐ Ⓑ Ⓒ Ⓓ   18. Ⓐ Ⓑ Ⓒ Ⓓ   28. Ⓐ Ⓑ Ⓒ Ⓓ

9. Ⓐ Ⓑ Ⓒ Ⓓ   19. Ⓐ Ⓑ Ⓒ Ⓓ   29. Ⓐ Ⓑ Ⓒ Ⓓ

10. Ⓐ Ⓑ Ⓒ Ⓓ   20. Ⓐ Ⓑ Ⓒ Ⓓ   30. Ⓐ Ⓑ Ⓒ Ⓓ

Answer Sheet – Part III – Reading Comprehension

1. (A) (B) (C) (D)   11. (A) (B) (C) (D)   21. (A) (B) (C) (D)   31. (A) (B) (C) (D)

2. (A) (B) (C) (D)   12. (A) (B) (C) (D)   22. (A) (B) (C) (D)   32. (A) (B) (C) (D)

3. (A) (B) (C) (D)   13. (A) (B) (C) (D)   23. (A) (B) (C) (D)   33. (A) (B) (C) (D)

4. (A) (B) (C) (D)   14. (A) (B) (C) (D)   24. (A) (B) (C) (D)   34. (A) (B) (C) (D)

5. (A) (B) (C) (D)   15. (A) (B) (C) (D)   25. (A) (B) (C) (D)   35. (A) (B) (C) (D)

6. (A) (B) (C) (D)   16. (A) (B) (C) (D)   26. (A) (B) (C) (D)

7. (A) (B) (C) (D)   17. (A) (B) (C) (D)   27. (A) (B) (C) (D)

8. (A) (B) (C) (D)   18. (A) (B) (C) (D)   28. (A) (B) (C) (D)

9. (A) (B) (C) (D)   19. (A) (B) (C) (D)   29. (A) (B) (C) (D)

10. (A) (B) (C) (D)   20. (A) (B) (C) (D)   30. (A) (B) (C) (D)

Answer Sheet – Part IV - Natural Sciences

1. Ⓐ Ⓑ Ⓒ Ⓓ   21. Ⓐ Ⓑ Ⓒ Ⓓ   41. Ⓐ Ⓑ Ⓒ Ⓓ

2. Ⓐ Ⓑ Ⓒ Ⓓ   22. Ⓐ Ⓑ Ⓒ Ⓓ   42. Ⓐ Ⓑ Ⓒ Ⓓ

3. Ⓐ Ⓑ Ⓒ Ⓓ   23. Ⓐ Ⓑ Ⓒ Ⓓ   43. Ⓐ Ⓑ Ⓒ Ⓓ

4. Ⓐ Ⓑ Ⓒ Ⓓ   24. Ⓐ Ⓑ Ⓒ Ⓓ   44. Ⓐ Ⓑ Ⓒ Ⓓ

5. Ⓐ Ⓑ Ⓒ Ⓓ   25. Ⓐ Ⓑ Ⓒ Ⓓ   45. Ⓐ Ⓑ Ⓒ Ⓓ

6. Ⓐ Ⓑ Ⓒ Ⓓ   26. Ⓐ Ⓑ Ⓒ Ⓓ   46. Ⓐ Ⓑ Ⓒ Ⓓ

7. Ⓐ Ⓑ Ⓒ Ⓓ   27. Ⓐ Ⓑ Ⓒ Ⓓ   47. Ⓐ Ⓑ Ⓒ Ⓓ

8. Ⓐ Ⓑ Ⓒ Ⓓ   28. Ⓐ Ⓑ Ⓒ Ⓓ   48. Ⓐ Ⓑ Ⓒ Ⓓ

9. Ⓐ Ⓑ Ⓒ Ⓓ   29. Ⓐ Ⓑ Ⓒ Ⓓ   49. Ⓐ Ⓑ Ⓒ Ⓓ

10. Ⓐ Ⓑ Ⓒ Ⓓ   30. Ⓐ Ⓑ Ⓒ Ⓓ   50. Ⓐ Ⓑ Ⓒ Ⓓ

11. Ⓐ Ⓑ Ⓒ Ⓓ   31. Ⓐ Ⓑ Ⓒ Ⓓ   51. Ⓐ Ⓑ Ⓒ Ⓓ

12. Ⓐ Ⓑ Ⓒ Ⓓ   32. Ⓐ Ⓑ Ⓒ Ⓓ   52. Ⓐ Ⓑ Ⓒ Ⓓ

13. Ⓐ Ⓑ Ⓒ Ⓓ   33. Ⓐ Ⓑ Ⓒ Ⓓ   53. Ⓐ Ⓑ Ⓒ Ⓓ

14. Ⓐ Ⓑ Ⓒ Ⓓ   34. Ⓐ Ⓑ Ⓒ Ⓓ   54. Ⓐ Ⓑ Ⓒ Ⓓ

15. Ⓐ Ⓑ Ⓒ Ⓓ   35. Ⓐ Ⓑ Ⓒ Ⓓ   55. Ⓐ Ⓑ Ⓒ Ⓓ

16. Ⓐ Ⓑ Ⓒ Ⓓ   36. Ⓐ Ⓑ Ⓒ Ⓓ   56. Ⓐ Ⓑ Ⓒ Ⓓ

17. Ⓐ Ⓑ Ⓒ Ⓓ   37. Ⓐ Ⓑ Ⓒ Ⓓ   57. Ⓐ Ⓑ Ⓒ Ⓓ

18. Ⓐ Ⓑ Ⓒ Ⓓ   38. Ⓐ Ⓑ Ⓒ Ⓓ   58. Ⓐ Ⓑ Ⓒ Ⓓ

19. Ⓐ Ⓑ Ⓒ Ⓓ   39. Ⓐ Ⓑ Ⓒ Ⓓ   59. Ⓐ Ⓑ Ⓒ Ⓓ

20. Ⓐ Ⓑ Ⓒ Ⓓ   40. Ⓐ Ⓑ Ⓒ Ⓓ   60. Ⓐ Ⓑ Ⓒ Ⓓ

Part 1 – Academic Aptitude

Vocabulary Sub-test

Directions: For each question below, select the word that is most different in meaning.

1. a. Torture b. Martyr c. Excruciate d. Torment

2. a. Quip b. Joke c. Jest d. Jaunty

3. a. Lodge b. Accommodate c. Billet d. Reside

4. a. Radiate b. Stellate c. Emanate d. Conciliate

5. a. Coquette b. Philander c. Romance d. Rebuff

6. a. Quixotic b. Romantic c. Amorous d. Loving

7. a. Lugubrious b. Languid c. Slow d. Laborious

8. a. Renegotiate b. Reconcile c. Harmonize d. Conciliate

9. a. Sanction b. Authorize c. Proscribe d. Approve

10. a. Progenitor b. Ancestor c. Antecedent d. Descendant

11. a. Conformist b. Iconoclast c. Maverick d. Unorthodox

12. a. Indolence b. Laziness c. Lugubrious d. Cheerful

13. a. Vulgar b. Decent c. Tasteless d. Brash

14. a. Unrelenting b. Ceaseless c. Constant d. Intermittent

15. a. Derision b. Scornful c. Approval d. Approbation

16. a. Roguishly b. Truthfully c. Dishonorably d. Disloyally

17. a. Giddiness b. Light-headedness c. Vertigo d. Phobia

18. a. Persistent b. Docile c. Pertinacious d. Tenacious

19. a. Boisterous b. Placid c. Rambunctious d. Rumbustious

20. a. Specious b. Spurious c. Legitimate d. Inauthentic

21. a. Invidious b. Discriminatory c. Unfavorable d. Apprehensible

22. a. Osculate b. Share c. Kiss d. Defalcate

23. a. Lie b. Veracity c. Mendacity d. Truth

24. a. Facet b. Feature c. Angle d. Whole

25. a. Negligent b. Discerning c. Prescient d. Discriminating

26. a. Venerate b. Esteem c. Disdain d. Prize

27. a. Redeemable b. Corrigible c. Amendable d. Catharsis

28. a. Raucous b. Noisy c. Orderly d. Obstreperous

29. a. Averse b. Loath c. Antipathetic d. Agreeable

30. a. Rampant b. Controlled c. Uncontrolled d. Abundant

Mathematics Sub-test

1. What is 1/3 of 3/4?

    a. 1/4
    b. 1/3
    c. 2/3
    d. 3/4

2. Susan wants to buy a leather jacket that costs $545.00 and is on sale for 10% off. What is the approximate cost?

    a. $525
    b. $450
    c. $475
    d. $500

3. 3.14 + 2.73 + 23.7 =

    a. 28.57
    b. 30.57
    c. 29.56
    d. 29.57

4. Express 0.27 + 0.33 as a fraction.

    a. 3/6
    b. 4/7
    c. 3/5
    d. 2/7

5. A woman spent 15% of her income on an item and ends up with $120. What percentage of her income is left?

    a. 12%

    b. 85%

    c. 75%

    d. 95%

6. 8 is what percent of 40?

    a. 10%

    b. 15%

    c. 20%

    d. 25%

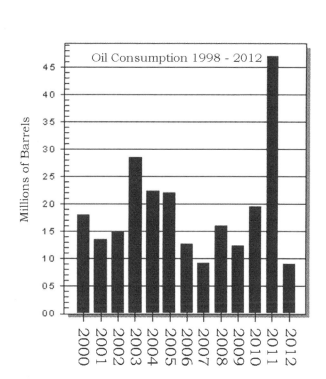

7. The graph above shows oil consumption in millions of barrels for the period, 1998 - 2012. What year did oil consumption peak?

    a. 2011

    b. 2010

    c. 2008

    d. 2009

8. Translate the following into an equation: 2 + a number divided by 7.

    a. (2 + X)/7
    b. (7 + X)/2
    c. (2 + 7)/X
    d. 2/(7 + X)

9. .4% of 36 is

    a. 1.44
    b. .144
    c. 14.4
    d. 144

10. The physician ordered 5 mg Coumadin; 10 mg/tablet is on hand. How many tablets will you give?

    a. .5 tablet
    b. 1 tablet
    c. .75 tablet
    d. 1.5 tablets

11. The physician ordered 20 mg Tylenol/kg of body weight; on hand is 80 mg/tablet. The child weighs 12 kg. How many tablets will you give?

    a. 1 tablet
    b. 3 tablets
    c. 2 tablets
    d. 4 tablets

12. What number is MCMXC?

    a. 1990
    b. 1980
    c. 2000
    d. 1995

13. Consider the following population growth chart.

Country	Population 2000	Population 2005
Japan	122,251,000	128,057,000
China	1,145,195,000	1,341,335,000
United States	253,339,000	310,384,000
Indonesia	184,346,000	239,871,000

What country is growing the fastest?

   a. Japan

   b. China

   c. United States

   d. Indonesia

14. If y = 4 and x = 3, solve yx^3

   a. -108

   b. 108

   c. 27

   d. 4

15. Convert 16 quarts to gallons.

   a. 1 gallons

   b. 8 gallons

   c. 4 gallons

   d. 4.5 gallons

16. Convert 45 kg. to pounds.

   a. 10 pounds

   b. 100 pounds

   c. 1,000 pounds

   d. 110 pounds

17. Translate the following into an equation: three plus a number times 7 equals 42.

    a. $7(3 + X) = 42$
    b. $3(X + 7) = 42$
    c. $3X + 7 = 42$
    d. $(3 + 7)X = 42$

18. In a class of 83 students, 72 are present. What percent of the students are absent? Provide answer up to two significant digits.

    a. 12%
    b. 13%
    c. 14%
    d. 15%

19. $5x+2(x+7) = 14x - 7$. Find x

    a. 1
    b. 2
    c. 3
    d. 4

20. $5(z+1) = 3(z+2) + 11$. Z=?

    a. 2
    b. 4
    c. 6
    d. 12

21. The price of a book went up from $20 to $25. What percent did the price increase?

    a. 5%
    b. 10%
    c. 20%
    d. 25%

22. A boy is given 2 apples while his sister is given 8 oranges. What is the ratio between the boy's apples and her oranges?

    a. 1:2

    b. 2:4

    c. 1:4

    d. 2:1

23. In the time required to serve 43 customers, a server breaks 2 glasses and slips 5 times. The next day, the same server breaks 10 glasses. How many customers did she serve?

    a. 25

    b. 43

    c. 86

    d. 215

24. A square lawn has an area of 62,500 square meters. What is the cost of building fence around it at a rate of $5.5 per meter?

    a. $4000

    b. $4500

    c. $5000

    d. $5500

25. Solve for n, when 5n + (19 – 2) = 67.

    a. 21

    b. 10

    c. 15

    d. 7

26. Below is the attendance for a class of 45.

Day	Number of Absent Students
Monday	5
Tuesday	9
Wednesday	4
Thursday	10
Friday	6

What is the average attendance for the week?

    a. 88%

    b. 85%

    c. 81%

    d. 77%

27. A distributor purchased 550 kilograms of potatoes for $165. He distributed these at a rate of $6.4 per 20 kilograms to 15 shops, $3.4 per 10 kilograms to 12 shops and the remainder at $1.8 per 5 kilograms. If his total distribution cost is $10, what will his profit be?

    a. $8.60

    b. $24.60

    c. $14.90

    d. $23.40

28. How much pay does Mr. Johnson receive if he gives half of his pay to his family, $250 to his landlord, and has exactly 3/7 of his pay left over?

    a. $3600

    b. $3500

    c. $2800

    d. $1750

29. A boy has 4 red, 5 green and 2 yellow balls. He chooses two balls randomly. What is the probability that one is red and other is green?

    a. 2/11

    b. 19/22

    c. 20/121

    d. 9/11

30. The cost of waterproofing canvas is .50 a square yard. What's the total cost for waterproofing a canvas truck cover that is 15' x 24'?

    a. $18.00

    b. $6.67

    c. $180.00

    d. $20.00

Nonverbal Sub-test

1.

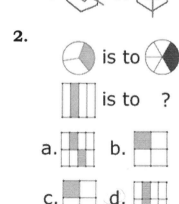

2.

3. 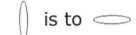 is to ⬯

△ is to ?

a. ▷   b. ◈

c. ◈   d. ◁

4. ⬚ is to ⬡

⬚ is to ?

a. ⬠   b. ⬡

c. ▢   d. △

5. ⬜ is to ◼

△ is to ?

a. ⬠   b. ▲

c. △   d. ⬡

6. ⬜ is to ▢⬠

⬠ is to ?

a. ⬠⬡   b. ▢⬡

c. ⬠⬡   d. ⬡⬡

7.

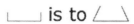 is to ⟋▽⟍

⟍▽⟍ is to ?

a. ⟋▽⟍ b. ⟋▽⟍

c. ⟍▽ d. ⟋▽⟍

8.

▢ is to ⌐|

⬠ is to ?

a. ⟩ b. ⟩

c. ⟩ d. ⏋

9.

☐ is to ⏋

⬠ is to ?

a. ⟩ b. ⟩

c. ⟩ d. ⏋

10. Consider the following sequence:

+ * + * | * + * + | * * + * | + + __ __

    a.   + *
    b. * *
    c. + +
    d. * +

Directions: Choose the option that completes a relationship that is the same as the relationship in the first pair.

11. Acting : Theater :: Gambling :

    a. Gym

    b. Bar

    c. Club

    d. Casino

12. Pork : Pig :: Beef :

    a. Herd

    b. Farmer

    c. Cow

    d. Lamb

13. Fruit : Banana :: Mammal :

    a. Cow

    b. Snake

    c. Fish

    d. Sparrow

14. Slumber : Sleep :: Bog :

    a. Dream

    b. Foray

    c. Swamp

    d. Night

15. Zoology : Animals

    a. Ecology : Pollution

    b. Botany : Plants

    c. Chemistry : Atoms

    d. History : People

16. Child : Human

    a. Dog : Pet

    b. Kitten : Cat

    c. Cow : Milk

    d. Bird : Robin

17. Wax : Candle

    a. Ink : Pen

    b. Clay : Bowl

    c. String : Kite

    d. Liquid : Cup

18. Which word does not belong with the others?

    a. Jet

    b. Float plane

    c. Kite

    d. Biplane

19. Which of the following does not belong?

    a. Number

    b. Denominate

    c. Numerate

    d. Figure

20. Which of the following does not belong?

    a. Abc

    b. bCD

    c. Nmo

    d. Pqr

21. Which of the following does not belong?

   a. CD
   b. OP
   c. LM
   d. BD

22. Which of the following does not belong?

   a. 121212
   b. 141414
   c. 151415
   d. 292929

23. Which of the following does not belong?

   a. 246
   b. 123
   c. 468
   d. 024

24. Which of the following does not belong?

   a. QRS
   b. LMN
   c. ACF
   d. RST

25. Which of the following does not belong?

   a. aBCd
   b. lMNo
   c. PQRs
   d. tUVw

26. Which of the following does not belong?

    a. ABCD

    b. JKLM

    c. PQRS

    d. WXYZ

27. Which of the following does not belong?

    a. BBCCDDEE

    b. LLMMNNOO

    c. HHIIJJKK

    d. RRSSTTUU

28. Which of the following does not belong?

    a. 123

    b. 246

    c. 456

    d. 789

29. Which of the following does not belong?

    a. def

    b. nop

    c. tuv

    d. lmn

30. Which of the following does not belong?

    a. Argue

    b. Talk

    c. Dispute

    d. Contest

Part II – Spelling

1. Choose the correct spelling.

    a. Realy

    b. Reelly

    c. Really

    d. None of the Above

2. Choose the correct spelling.

    a. Rescede

    b. Receede

    c. Reacede

    d. Recede

3. Choose the correct spelling.

    a. Refrense

    b. Refrence

    c. Reference

    d. Refference

4. Choose the correct spelling.

    a. Similar

    b. Similiar

    c. Simillar

    d. Semilar

5. Choose the correct spelling.

    a. Sking

    b. Skying

    c. Skiing

    d. Skinng

6. Choose the correct spelling.

    a. Stregth

    b. Stregth

    c. Strength

    d. Strenth

7. Choose the correct spelling.

    a. Technical

    b. Tecknical

    c. Techical

    d. Teknical

8. Choose the correct spelling.

    a. Theries

    b. Theories

    c. Theorys

    d. Theorries

9. Choose the correct spelling.

    a. Possess

    b. Posese

    c. Posess

    d. Poses

10. Choose the correct spelling.

    a. Portrey

    b. Portray

    c. Potray

    d. Porttray

11. Choose the correct spelling.

    a. Proceadure

    b. Proceedure

    c. Procedure

    d. Procedrure

12. Choose the correct spelling.

    a. Proceed

    b. Proced

    c. Procead

    d. Procceed

13. Choose the correct spelling.

    a. Profresor

    b. Proffessor

    c. Profesor

    d. Professor

14. Choose the correct spelling.

    a. Persue

    b. Pursu

    c. Pursue

    d. Porsue

15. Choose the correct spelling.

    a. Realice

    b. Realize

    c. Relise

    d. None of the Above

16. Choose the correct spelling.

    a. Peice

    b. Pece

    c. Piece

    d. Peece

17. Choose the correct spelling.

    a. Posibel

    b. Posible

    c. Possible

    d. None of the Above

18. Choose the correct spelling.

    a. Encouraging

    b. Encuraging

    c. Encuoraging

    d. None of the Above

19. Choose the correct spelling.

    a. Harras

    b. Harasse

    c. Harass

    d. Haress

20. Choose the correct spelling.

    a. Manetain

    b. Maintain

    c. Maintane

    d. Manetane

21. Choose the correct spelling.

    a. Hieght

    b. Height

    c. Heit

    d. Heigt

22. Choose the correct spelling.

    a. Heross

    b. Heros

    c. Herose

    d. Heroes

23. Choose the correct spelling.

    a. Geneus

    b. Genius

    c. Ginius

    d. Gennius

24. Choose the correct spelling.

    a. Incedentally

    b. Incidentaly

    c. Incidentally

    d. Incidentilly

25. Choose the correct spelling.

    a. Parallel

    b. Parallell

    c. Paralel

    d. Parralel

26. Choose the correct spelling.

    a. Absenes

    b. Absence

    c. Absense

    d. Absennce

27. Choose the correct spelling.

    a. Advurtisement

    b. Advertisment

    c. Advertisement

    d. Advertesement

28. Choose the correct spelling.

    a. Bileif

    b. Bilief

    c. Beleif

    d. Belief

29. Choose the correct spelling.

    a. Comparative

    b. Comperative

    c. Comparetive

    d. Conparative

30. Choose the correct spelling.

    a. Definately

    b. Definitely

    c. Definetely

    d. Difenitely

Reading Comprehension.

Questions 1 – 4 refer to the following passage.

Passage 1 - Infectious Disease

An infectious disease is a clinically evident illness resulting from the presence of pathogenic agents, such as viruses, bacteria, fungi, protozoa, multi-cellular parasites, and unusual proteins known as prions. Infectious pathologies are also called communicable diseases or transmissible diseases, due to their potential of transmission from one person or species to another by a replicating agent (as opposed to a toxin).

Transmission of an infectious disease can occur in many different ways. Physical contact, liquids, food, body fluids, contaminated objects, and airborne inhalation can all transmit infecting agents.

Transmissible diseases that occur through contact with an ill person, or objects touched by them, are especially infective, and are sometimes called contagious diseases. Communicable diseases that require a more specialized route of infection, such as through blood or needle transmission, or sexual transmission, are usually not regarded as contagious.

The term infectivity describes the ability of an organism to enter, survive and multiply in the host, while the infectiousness of a disease indicates the comparative ease with which the disease is transmitted. An infection however, is not synonymous with an infectious disease, as an infection may not cause important clinical symptoms. [9]

1. What can we infer from the first paragraph in this passage?

a. Sickness from a toxin can be easily transmitted from one person to another.

b. Sickness from an infectious disease can be easily transmitted from one person to another.

c. Few sicknesses are transmitted from one person to another.

d. Infectious diseases are easily treated.

2. What are two other names for infections' pathologies?

a. Communicable diseases or transmissible diseases

b. Communicable diseases or terminal diseases

c. Transmissible diseases or preventable diseases

d. Communicative diseases or unstable diseases

3. What does infectivity describe?

a. The inability of an organism to multiply in the host

b. The inability of an organism to reproduce

c. The ability of an organism to enter, survive and multiply in the host

d. The ability of an organism to reproduce in the host

4. How do we know an infection is not synonymous with an infectious disease?

a. Because an infectious disease destroys infections with enough time.

b. Because an infection may not cause important clinical symptoms or impair host function.

c. We do not. The two are synonymous.

d. Because an infection is too fatal to be an infectious disease.

Questions 5 – 8 refer to the following passage.

Passage 2 - Virus

A virus (from the Latin virus meaning toxin or poison) is a small infectious agent that can replicate only inside the living cells of other organisms. Most viruses are too small to be seen directly with a microscope. Viruses infect all types of organisms, from animals and plants to bacteria and single-celled organisms.

Unlike prions and viroids, viruses consist of two or three parts: all viruses have genes made from either DNA or RNA, all have a protein coat that protects these genes, and some have an envelope of fat that surrounds them when they are outside a cell. (Viroids do not have a protein coat and prions contain no RNA or DNA.) Viruses vary from simple to very complex structures. Most viruses are about one hundred times smaller than an average bacterium. The origins of viruses in the evolutionary history of life are unclear: some may have evolved from plasmids—pieces of DNA that can move between cells—while others may have evolved from bacteria.

Viruses spread in many ways; plant viruses are often transmitted from plant to plant by insects that feed on sap, such as aphids, while animal viruses can be carried by blood-sucking insects. These disease-bearing organisms are known as vectors. Influenza viruses are spread by coughing and sneezing. HIV is one of several viruses transmitted through sexual contact and by exposure to infected blood. Viruses can infect only a limited range of host cells called the "host range." This can be broad as, when a virus is capable of infecting many species or narrow. [10]

5. What can we infer from the first paragraph in this selection?

  a. A virus is the same as bacterium

  b. A person with excellent vision can see a virus with the naked eye

  c. A virus cannot be seen with the naked eye

  d. Not all viruses are dangerous

6. What types of organisms do viruses infect?

  a. Only plants and humans

  b. Only animals and humans

  c. Only disease-prone humans

  d. All types of organisms

7. How many parts do prions and viroids consist of?

  a. Two

  b. Three

  c. Either less than two or more than three

  d. Less than two

8. What is one common virus spread by coughing and sneezing?

  a. AIDS

  b. Influenza

  c. Herpes

  d. Tuberculosis

Questions 9 – 11 refer to the following passage.

Passage 3 – Thunderstorms

The first stage of a thunderstorm is the cumulus stage, or developing stage. In this stage, masses of moisture are lifted upwards into the atmosphere. The trigger for this lift can be insulation heating the ground producing thermals, areas where two winds converge, forcing air upwards, or where winds blow over terrain of increasing elevation. Moisture in the air rapidly cools into liquid drops of water, which appears as cumulus clouds.

As the water vapor condenses into liquid, latent heat is released which warms the air, causing it to become less dense than the surrounding dry air. The warm air rises in an updraft through the process of convection (hence the term convective precipitation). This creates a low-pressure zone beneath the forming thunderstorm. In a typical thunderstorm, about 5×10^8 kg of water vapor is lifted, and the quantity of energy released when this condenses is about equal to the energy used by a city of 100,000 in a month. [11]

9. The cumulus stage of a thunderstorm is the

    a. The last stage of the storm

    b. The middle stage of the storm formation

    c. The beginning of the thunderstorm

    d. The period after the thunderstorm has ended

10. One of the ways the air is warmed is

    a. Air moving downwards, which creates a high-pressure zone

    b. Air cooling and becoming less dense, causing it to rise

    c. Moisture moving downward toward the earth

    d. Heat created by water vapor condensing into liquid

11. Identify the correct sequence of events

    a. Warm air rises, water droplets condense, creating more heat, and the air rises farther.

    b. Warm air rises and cools, water droplets condense, causing low pressure.

    c. Warm air rises and collects water vapor, the water vapor condenses as the air rises, which creates heat, and causes the air to rise farther.

    d. None of the above.

Questions 12 – 14 refer to the following passage.

Passage 4 – US Weather Service

The United States National Weather Service classifies thunderstorms as severe when they reach a predetermined level. Usually, this means the storm is strong enough to inflict wind or hail damage. In most of the United States, a storm is considered severe if winds reach over 50 knots (58 mph or 93 km/h), hail is ¾ inch (2 cm) diameter or larger, or if meteorologists report funnel clouds or tornadoes. In the Central Region of the United States National Weather Service, the hail threshold for a severe thunderstorm is 1 inch (2.5 cm) in diameter. Though a funnel cloud or tornado indicates the presence of a severe thunderstorm, the various meteorological agencies would issue a tornado warning rather than a severe thunderstorm warning.

Meteorologists in Canada define a severe thunderstorm as either having tornadoes, wind gusts of 90 km/h or greater, hail 2 centimeters in diameter or greater, rainfall more than 50 millimeters in 1 hour, or 75 millimeters in 3 hours.

Severe thunderstorms can develop from any type of thunderstorm. [12]

12. What is the purpose of this passage?

a. Explaining when a thunderstorm turns into a tornado

b. Explaining who issues storm warnings, and when these warnings should be issued

c. Explaining when meteorologists consider a thunderstorm severe

d. None of the above

13. It is possible to infer from this passage that

a. Different areas and countries have different criteria for determining a severe storm

b. Thunderstorms can include lightning and tornadoes, as well as violent winds and large hail

c. If someone spots both a thunderstorm and a tornado, meteorological agencies will immediately issue a severe storm warning

d. Canada has a much different alert system for severe storms, with criteria that are far less

14. What would the Central Region of the United States National Weather Service do if hail was 2.7 cm in diameter?

a. Not issue a severe thunderstorm warning.

b. Issue a tornado warning.

c. Issue a severe thunderstorm warning.

d. Sleet must also accompany the hail before the Weather Service will issue a storm warning.

Question 15 refers to the following Table of Contents.

Contents

15. Consider the table of contents above. What page would you find information about natural selection and adaptation?

a. 81

b. 90

c. 110

d. 132

Questions 16 – 19 refer to the following passage.

Passage 5 – Clouds

A cloud is a visible mass of droplets or frozen crystals floating in the atmosphere above the surface of the Earth or other planetary bodies. Another type of cloud is a mass of material in space, attracted by gravity, called interstellar clouds and nebulae. The branch of meteorology which studies clouds is called nephrology. When we are speaking of Earth clouds, water vapor is usually the condensing substance, which forms small droplets or ice crystal. These crystals are typically 0.01 mm in diameter. Dense, deep clouds reflect most light, so they appear white, at least from the top. Cloud droplets scatter light very efficiently, so the farther into a cloud light travels, the weaker it gets. This accounts for the gray or dark appearance at the base of large clouds. Thin clouds may appear to have acquired the color of their environment or background. [12]

16. What are clouds made of?

a. Water droplets.

b. Ice crystals.

c. Ice crystals and water droplets.

d. Clouds on Earth are made of ice crystals and water droplets.

17. The main idea of this passage is

a. Condensation occurs in clouds, having an intense effect on the weather on the surface of the earth.

b. Atmospheric gases are responsible for the gray color of clouds just before a severe storm happens.

c. A cloud is a visible mass of droplets or frozen crystals floating in the atmosphere above the surface of the Earth or other planetary body.

d. Clouds reflect light in varying amounts and degrees, depending on the size and concentration of the water droplets.

18. The branch of meteorology that studies clouds is called

a. Convection

b. Thermal meteorology

c. Nephology

d. Nephelometry

19. Why are clouds white on top and grey on the bottom?

a. Because water droplets inside the cloud do not reflect light, it appears white, and the farther into the cloud the light travels, the less light is reflected making the bottom appear dark.

b. Because water droplets outside the cloud reflect light, it appears dark, and the farther into the cloud the light travels, the more light is reflected making the bottom appear white.

c. Because water droplets inside the cloud reflects light, making it appear white, and the farther into the cloud the light travels, the more light is reflected making the bottom appear dark.

d. None of the above.

Questions 20 - 23 refer to the following recipe.

Who Was Anne Frank?

You may have heard mention of the word Holocaust in your History or English classes. The Holocaust took place from 1939-1945. It was an attempt by the Nazi party to purify the human race, by eliminating Jews, Gypsies, Catholics, homosexuals and others they deemed inferior to their "perfect" Aryan race. The Nazis used Concentration Camps, which were sometimes used as Death Camps, to exterminate the people they held in the camps. One of the saddest facts about the Holocaust was the over one million children under the age of sixteen died in a Nazi concentration camp. Just a few weeks before World War II was over, Anne Frank was one of those children to die.

Before the Nazi party began its persecution of the Jews, Anne Frank had a happy live. She was born in June of 1929. In June of 1942, for her 13th birthday, she was given a simple present which would go onto impact the lives of millions of people around the world. That gift was a small red diary that she called Kitty. This diary was to become Anne's most treasured possession when she and her family hid from the Nazi's in a secret annex above her father's office building in Amsterdam.

For 25 months, Anne, her sister Margot, her parents, another family, and an elderly Jewish dentist hid from the Nazis in this tiny annex. They were never permitted to go outside, and their food and supplies were brought to them by Miep Gies and her husband, who did not believe in the Nazi persecution of the Jews. It was a very difficult life for young Anne and she used Kitty as an outlet to describe her life in hiding.

After 2 years, Anne and her family were betrayed and arrested by the Nazis. To this day, nobody is exactly sure who betrayed the Frank family and the other annex residents. Anne, her mother, and her sister were separated from Otto Frank, Anne's father. Then, Anne and Margot were separated from their mother. In March of 1945, Margot Frank died of starvation in a Concentration Camp. A few days later, at the age of 15, Anne Frank died of typhus. Of all the people who hid in the Annex, only Otto Frank survived the Holocaust.

Otto Frank returned to the Annex after World War II. It was there that he found Kitty, filled with Anne's thoughts and feelings about being a persecuted Jewish girl. Otto Frank had Anne's diary published in 1947 and it has remained continuously in print ever since. Today, the diary has been published in over 55 languages and more than 24 million copies have been sold around the world. The Diary of Anne Frank tells the story of a brave young woman who tried to see the good in all people.

20. From the context clues in the passage, the word Annex most nearly means?

    a. Attic

    b. Bedroom

    c. Basement

    d. Kitchen

21. Why do you think Anne's diary has been published in 55 languages?

    a. So everyone could understand it.

    b. So people around the world could learn more about the horrors of the Holocaust.

    c. Because Anne was Jewish but hid in Amsterdam and died in Germany.

    d. Because Otto Frank spoke many languages.

22. From the description of Anne and Margot's deaths in the passage, what can we assume typhus is?

    a. The same as starving to death.

    b. An infection the Germans gave to Anne.

    c. A disease Anne caught in the concentration camp.

    d. Poison gas used by the Germans to kill Anne.

23. In the third paragraph, what does the word outlet most nearly mean?

    a. A place to plug things into the wall

    b. A store where Miep bought cheap supplies for the Frank family

    c. A hiding space similar to an Annex

    d. A place where Anne could express her private thoughts.

Questions 24 – 25 refer to the following email.

SUBJECT: MEDICAL STAFF CHANGES

To all staff:

This email is to advise you of a paper on recommended medical staff changes has been posted to the Human Resources website.

The contents are of primary interest to medical staff, other staff may be interested in reading it, particularly those in medical support roles.

The paper deals with several major issues:

    1. Improving our ability to attract top quality staff to the hospital, and retain our existing staff. These changes will make our position and departmental names internationally recognizable and comparable with North American and North Asian departments and positions.

    2. Improving our ability to attract top quality staff by introducing greater flexibility in the departmental structure.

    3. General comments on issues to be further discussed in relation to research staff.

The changes outlined in this paper are significant. I encourage you to read the document and send to me any comments you may have, so that it can be enhanced and improved.

Gordon Simms
Administrator,
Seven Oaks Regional Hospital

24. Are all hospital staff required to read the document posted to the Human Resources website?

    a. Yes all staff are required to read the document.

    b. No, reading the document is optional.

    c. Only medical staff are required to read the document.

    d. none of the above are correct.

25. Have the changes to medical staff been made?

    a. Yes, the changes have been made.

    b. No, the changes are only being discussed.

    c. Some of the changes have been made.

    d. None of the choices are correct.

Questions 26 – 29 refer to the following passage.

Passage 6 – Navy Seals

The United States Navy's Sea, Air and Land Teams, commonly known as Navy SEALs, are the U.S. Navy's principle special operations force, and a part of the Naval Special Warfare Command (NSWC) as well as the maritime component of the United States Special Operations Command (USSOCOM).

The unit's acronym ("SEAL") comes from their capacity to operate at sea, in the air, and on land – but it is their ability to work underwater that separates SEALs from most other military units in the world. Navy SEALs are trained and have been deployed in a wide variety of missions, including direct action and special reconnaissance operations, unconventional warfare, foreign internal defence, hostage rescue, counter-terrorism and other missions. All SEALs are members of either the United States Navy or the United States Coast Guard.

In the early morning of May 2, 2011 local time, a team of 40 CIA-led Navy SEALs completed an operation to kill Osama bin Laden in Abbottabad, Pakistan about 35 miles (56 km) from Islamabad, the country's capital. The Navy SEALs were part of the Naval Special Warfare Development Group, previously called "Team 6." President Barack Obama later confirmed the death of bin Laden. The unprecedented media coverage raised the public profile of the SEAL community, particularly the counter-terrorism specialists commonly known as SEAL Team 6. [13]

26. Are Navy SEALs part of USSOCOM?

a. Yes

b. No

c. Only for special operations

d. No, they are part of the US Navy

27. What separates Navy SEALs from other military units?

a. Belonging to NSWC

b. Direct action and special reconnaissance operations

c. Working underwater

d. Working for other military units in the world

28. What other military organizations do SEALs belong to?

a. The US Navy

b. The Coast Guard

c. The US Army

d. The Navy and the Coast Guard

29. What other organization participated in the Bin Laden raid?

a. The CIA

b. The US Military

c. Counter-terrorism specialists

d. None of the above

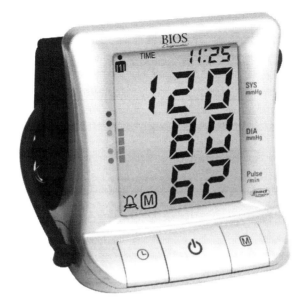

30. Consider the blood pressure gauge above. According to this gauge, what is the patient's pulse?

    a. 120 beats per minute

    b. 80 beats per minute

    c. 62 beats per minute

    d. The pulse is not shown

Questions 31 – 33 refer to the following passage.

Passage 7 - Was Dr. Seuss A Real Doctor?

A favorite author for over 100 years, Theodor Seuss Geisel was born on March 2, 1902. Today, we celebrate the birthday of the famous "Dr. Seuss" by hosting Read Across America events throughout the month of March. School children around the country celebrate the "Doctor's" birthday by making hats, giving presentations and holding read aloud circles featuring some of Dr. Seuss' most famous books.

But who was Dr. Seuss? Did he go to medical school? Where was his office? You may be surprised to know that Theodor Seuss Geisel was not a medical doctor at all. He took on the nickname Dr. Seuss when he became a noted children's book author. He earned the nickname because people said his books were "as good as medicine." All these years later, his nickname has lasted and he is known as Dr. Seuss all across the world.

Think back to when you were a young child. Did you ever want to try "green eggs and ham.?" Did you try to "Hop on Pop?" Do you remember learning about the environment from a creature called The Lorax? Of course, you must recall one of Seuss' most famous characters; that green Grinch who stole Christmas. These stories were all written by Dr. Seuss and featured his signature rhyming words and letters. They also featured made up words to enhance his rhyme scheme and even though many of his characters were made up, they sure seem real to us today.

And what of his "signature" book, The Cat in the Hat? You must remember that cat and Thing One and Thing Two from your childhood. Did you know that in the early 1950's there was a growing concern in America that children were not becoming avid readers? This was, book publishers thought, because children found books dull and uninteresting. An intelligent publisher sent Dr. Seuss a book of words that he thought all children should learn as young readers. Dr. Seuss wrote his famous story The Cat in the Hat, using those words. We can see, over the decades, just how much influence his writing has had on very young children. That is why we celebrate this doctor's birthday each March.

31. What does the word "avid" mean in the last paragraph?

    a. Good

    b. Interested

    c. Slow

    d. Fast

32. What can we infer from the statement " His books were like medicine?"

    a. His books made people feel better

    b. His books were in doctor's office waiting rooms

    c. His books took away fevers

    d. His books left a funny taste in readers' mouths.

33. Why is the publisher in the last paragraph referred to as "intelligent?"

a. The publisher knew how to read.

b. The publisher knew kids did not like to read.

c. The publisher knew Dr. Seuss would be able to create a book that sold well.

d. The publisher knew that Dr. Seuss would be able to write a book that would get young children interested in reading.

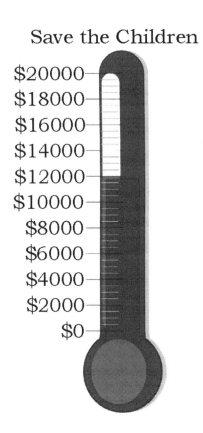

34. Consider the graphic above. The Save the Children fund has a fund-raising goal of $20,000. Approximately how much of their goal have they achieved?

a. 3/5

b. 3/4

c. 1/2

d. 1/3

35. Consider the graphic above. The Save the Children fund has a fund-raising goal of $16,000. Approximately how much of their goal have they achieved?

   a. 3/5

   b. 3/4

   c. 1/2

   d. 1/3

Section IV – Basic Science

1. Describe the differences between genotypes and phenotypes

   a. Phenotype refers to observed properties of an organism and genotype refers to the genes of an organism.

   b. Genotype refers to observed properties of an organism and phenotype refers to the genes of an organism.

   c. Phenotype refers to the DNA of an organism and genotype refers to the genes of an organism.

   d. Genotype refers to the DNA of an organism and phenotype refers to the genes of an organism.

2. A solution with a pH value of greater than 7 is

   a. Base

   b. Acid

   c. Neutral

   d. None of the above

3. Eukaryotic and prokaryotic cells are

   a. Both organelles

   b. Eukaryotic are not organelles

   c. Both have DNA

   d. Both have single membrane compartments

4. When we say that important traits for scientific classification are homologous, "homologous" means

    a. Being shared among two or more animals with the same parent.

    b. Being coincidentally shared by two totally different creatures.

    c. Being inherited by the organisms' common ancestors.

    d. Mutating beyond all reasonable expectations.

5. The manner in which instructions for building proteins, the basic structural molecules of living material, are written in the DNA is

    a. Genotypic assignment

    b. Chromosome pattern

    c. Genetic code

    d. Genetic fingerprinting

6. A _____ is a unit of inherited material, encoded by a strand of DNA and transcribed by RNA.

    a. Allele

    b. Phenotype

    c. Gene

    d. Genotype

7. Which, if any, of the following statements about meiosis are correct?

    a. During meiosis, the number of chromosomes in the cell are halved.

    b. Meiosis only occurs in eukaryotic cells.

    c. Meiosis is the part of the life cycle that involves sexual reproduction.

    d. All of these statements are correct.

8. A population of wolves expanded exponentially after a hunting ban. Within a few generations, their habitat exceeded its

    a. Carrying capacity

    b. Food source

    c. Population limit

    d. Supply capability

9. When a pouch in the large intestine becomes inflamed, this becomes an affliction known as

  a. Diverticulosis

  b. Diverticulitis

  c. Acid Reflux

  d. Colon Cancer

10. Why is detection of pathogens complicated?

  a. They evolve so quickly

  b. They die so quickly

  c. They are invisible

  d. They multiply so quickly

11. Photosynthesis is:

  a. The process by which plants generate oxygen from carbon dioxide.

  b. The process by which plants generate carbon dioxide from oxygen.

  c. The process by which plants generate carbon dioxide and oxygen.

  d. None of the above.

12. Which, if any, of the following statements are false?

  a. A mutation is a permanent change in the DNA sequence of a gene.

  b. Mutations in a gene's DNA sequence can alter the amino acid sequence of the protein encoded by the gene.

  c. Mutations in DNA sequences usually occur spontaneously.

  d. Mutations in DNA sequences can be caused by exposure to environmental agents such as sunshine.

13. Starting with the weakest, arrange the fundamental forces of nature in order of strength.

  a. Gravity, Weak Nuclear Force, Electromagnetic Force, Strong Nuclear Force

  b. Weak Nuclear Force, Gravity, Electromagnetic Force, Strong Nuclear Force

  c. Strong Nuclear Force, Weak Nuclear Force, Electromagnetic Force, Gravity

  d. Gravity, Strong Nuclear Force, Weak Nuclear Force, Electromagnetic Force

14. _____, **which refers to the repeatability of measurement, does not require knowledge of the correct or true value.**

    a. Precision

    b. Value

    c. Certainty

    d. Accuracy

15. Artificial selection:

    a. Is a process where desirable traits are systematically bred

    b. Is a process where traits become more or less common in a population

    c. Is a process where behaviors are favored

    d. None of the above.

16. Which of the following are not examples of vaporization?

    a. Boiling

    b. Evaporation

    c. Condensation

    d. All of the above

17. Describe the periodic table.

    a. The periodic table is a tabular display of the chemical compounds organized on the basis of their atomic numbers, electron configurations, and recurring chemical properties.

    b. The periodic table is a tabular display of the chemical elements, organized on the basis of their atomic numbers, electron configurations, and recurring chemical properties.

    c. The periodic table is a tabular display of the chemical subatomic particles, organized on the basis of their atomic numbers, electron configurations, and recurring chemical properties.

    d. None of the above.

18. In terms of the scientific method, the term _____ refers to the act of noticing or perceiving something and/or recording a fact or occurrence.

    a. Observation

    b. Diligence

    c. Perception

    d. Control

19. What is the difference, of any, between kinetic energy and potential energy?

    a. Kinetic energy is the energy of a body that results from heat while potential energy is the energy possessed by an object that is chilled

    b. Kinetic energy is the energy of a body that results from motion while potential energy is the energy possessed by an object by virtue of its position or state, e.g., as in a compressed spring.

    c. There is no difference between kinetic and potential energy; all energy is the same.

    d. Potential energy is the energy of a body that results from motion while kinetic energy is the energy possessed by an object by virtue of its position or state, e.g., as in a compressed spring.

20. What is the sequence of developmental stages through which members of a given species must pass?

    a. Life cycle

    b. Life expectancy

    c. Life sequence

    d. None of the above

21. Which one of the following best describes the function of a cell membrane?

    a. It controls the substances entering and leaving the cell.

    b. It keeps the cell in shape.

    c. It controls the substances entering the cell.

    d. It supports the cell structures

22. Which of these is not a rank within the area of classification or taxonomy?

    a. Species

    b. Family

    c. Genus

    d. Relative position

23. The scientific term _____ refers to a practical test designed with the intention that its results be relevant to a particular theory or set of theories.

    a. Procedure

    b. Variable

    c. Hypothesis

    d. Experiment

24. Substances that deactivate catalysts are called

    a. Inhibitors

    b. Catalytic poisons

    c. Positive catalysts

    d. None of the above

25. Describe kinetic energy.

    a. Kinetic energy is the energy an object possesses due to its mass.

    b. Kinetic energy is the energy an object possesses due to its motion.

    c. Kinetic energy is the energy an object possesses due to its chemical properties.

    d. Kinetic energy is the stored energy an object possesses.

26. The interval of confidence around the measured value such that the measured value is certain not to lie outside this stated interval refers to the _____ of that value.

    a. Accuracy

    b. Error

    c. Uncertainty

    d. Measurement

27. What are the differences, if any, between arteries, veins, and capillaries?

    a. Veins carry oxygenated blood away from the heart, arteries return oxygen-depleted blood to the heart, and capillaries are thin-walled blood vessels in which gas/ nutrient/ waste exchange occurs.

    b. Capillaries carry oxygenated blood away from the heart, veins return oxygen-depleted blood to the heart, and capillaries are thin-walled blood vessels in which gas/ nutrient/ waste exchange occurs.

    c. There are no differences; all perform the same function in different parts of the body.

    d. Arteries carry oxygenated blood away from the heart, veins return oxygen-depleted blood to the heart, and capillaries are thin-walled blood vessels in which gas/ nutrient/ waste exchange occurs.

28. What part of the body initiates inhalation?

    a. The lungs

    b. The diaphragm

    c. The larynx

    d. The kidneys

29. Another term for biological classification is:

    a. Darwinian classification.

    b. Animal classification.

    c. Molecular classification.

    d. Scientific classification.

30. What type of gene is not expressed as a trait unless inherited by both parents?

    a. Principal gene

    b. Latent gene

    c. Recessive gene

    d. Dominant gene

31. What is an approximation or simulation of a real system that omits all but the most essential variables of the system.

    a. Scientific method

    b. Independent variable

    c. Control group

    d. Scientific model

32. Neutrons are necessary within an atomic nucleus because:

    a. They bind with protons via nuclear force

    b. They bind with nuclei via nuclear force

    c. They bind with protons via electromagnetic force

    d. They bind with nuclei via electromagnetic force

33. Which of the following statements are false?

    a. Most enzymes are proteins

    b. Enzymes are catalysts

    c. Most enzymes are inorganic

    d. Enzymes are large biological molecules

34. _____ are compounds that contain hydrogen, can dissolve in water to release hydrogen ions into solution, and, in an aqueous solution, can conduct electricity.

    a. Caustics

    b. Bases

    c. Acids

    d. Salts

35. What are the basic structural units of nucleic acids (DNA or RNA) whose sequence determines individual hereditary characteristics?

    a. Gene

    b. Nucleotide

    c. Phosphate

    d. Nitrogen base

36. List the classifications of organisms in order of size.

    a. Genus, Kingdom, Phylum/division, Class, Order, and Family Species

    b. Order, Kingdom, Phylum/division, Genus, Class, and Family Species

    c. Genus, Kingdom, Phylum/division, Class, Order, and Family Species

    d. Kingdom ,Genus, Phylum/division, Class, Order, and Family Species

    e. Family species, Order, Class, Phylum/division, Kingdom, and Genus

37. Where does digestion begin?

    a. In the throat

    b. In the stomach

    c. In the intestines

    d. In the mouth

38. What are the main components of the circulatory system?

    a. The heart, veins and blood vessels

    b. The heart, brain, and ears

    c. The nose, throat and ears

    d. The lungs, stomach, and kidneys

39. What is an example of a pathogen that the immune system detects?

    a. An atom

    b. A molecule

    c. A vitamin

    d. A virus

40. Explain chemical bonds.

a. Chemical bonds are attractions between atoms that form chemical substances containing two or more atoms.

b. Chemical bonds are attractions between protons that form chemical elements containing two or more atoms.

c. Chemical bonds are two or more atoms that form chemical substances.

d. None of the above

41. Which of these is not an example of a function of the stomach in digestion?

a. Storing food

b. Cleansing food of impurities

c. Mixing food with digestive juices

d. Transferring food into the intestines

42. The exchange of oxygen for carbon dioxide takes place in the alveolar area of _____.

a. The throat

b. The ears

c. The appendix

d. The lungs

43. The number of protons in the nucleus of an atom is the

a. Atomic mass

b. Atomic weight

c. Atomic number

d. None of the above

44. Natural selection is:

a. A process where biological traits become more common in a population

b. A process where biological traits become less common in a population

c. A process where biological traits become more or less common in a population

d. None of the above

45. Sex chromosomes are designated as being "X" or "Y" chromosomes. In terms of sex chromosomes, what differences exist between males and females?

a. Females have two X chromosomes and males have one X chromosome and one Y chromosome.

b. Females have one X chromosome, and males have one X chromosome and one Y chromosome.

c. Females have one Y chromosome, while males have one X chromosome.

d. Females have one X chromosome and one Y chromosome, and males have two X chromosomes.

46. How does the immune system fight off disease?

a. By identifying and killing tumor cells and pathogens.

b. By creating new blood cells that fight disease.

c. By expelling infection through the blood stream.

d. By giving you energy to resist disease infections.

47. Identify the chemical properties of water.

a. Water has two hydrogen atoms covalently bonded to one oxygen atom

b. Water has two oxygen atoms covalently bonded to one hydrogen atom

c. Water has two hydrogen atoms polar covalently bonded to one oxygen atom

d. Water has two oxygen atoms polar covalently bonded to one hydrogen atom

48. Which of the following is not true of atomic theory?

a. Originated in the early 19th century with the work of John Dalton.

b. Is the field of physics that describes the characteristics and properties of atoms that make up matter.

c. Explains temperature as the momentum of atoms.

d. Explains macroscopic phenomenon through the behavior of microscopic atoms.

49. A condition in which the heart beats too fast, too slow, or with an irregular beat is called _____.

    a. Hypertension

    b. Angina

    c. Cardiac arrest

    d. Arrythmia

50. The best way to avoid most digestive diseases is _____.

    a. Eating a healthy diet

    b. Eating only proteins

    c. Never eating dessert

    d. Trying not to get angry

51. An example of an important side-benefit of the respiratory system is

    a. The air allows whistling.

    b. The oxygen expelled can be recycled for other uses.

    c. The air being expelled from the mouth allows for speaking.

    d. The air expelled from the body also expels disease and germs.

52. An example of a disease of the lungs that is caused or made worse by smoking is

    a. Emphysema

    b. Strep throat

    c. Muscular dystrophy

    d. Leukemia

53. What is an example of an early response by the immune system to infection?

    a. Inhalation

    b. Inflammation

    c. Respiration

    d. Exhalation

54. Which cells are an important weapon in the fight against infection?

  a. Red blood cells

  b. White blood cells

  c. Barrier cells

  d. Virus cells

55. The complementary bases found in DNA are _____ and _____ or _____ and _____.

  a. Adenine and thymine or cytosine and guanine

  b. Cytosine and thymine or adenine and guanine

  c. Adenine and cytosine or thymine and guanine

  d. None of the above

56. The full complement of genes carried by a single set of chromosomes is a _____.

  a. Genome

  b. Genetics

  c. Genetic code

  d. Gene amplification

57. _____ is a classification of organisms into different categories based on their physical characteristics and presumed natural relationship.

  a. Biology

  b. Taxonomy

  c. Grouping

  d. Nomenclature

57. What is the order of hierarchy of levels in the biological classification of organisms?

  a. Kingdom, phylum, class, order, family, genus, and species

  b. Phylum, kingdom, class, order, family, genus, and species

  c. Order, phylum, class, kingdom, family, genus, and species

  d. Kingdom, phylum, order, class, family, genus, and species

59. What is any compound produced by a chemical reaction between a base and an acid?

   a. Salt

   b. Radical

   c. Crystal

   d. Electrolyte

60. What is a graphical description of feeding relationships among species in an ecological community.

   a. Food web

   b. Food chain

   c. Food network

   d. Food sequence

Answer Key

Vocabulary

1. B

2. D

3. D

4. D

5. D

6. A

7. D

8. A

9. C

10. D

11. A

12. D

13. B

14. D

15. C

16. B

17. D

18. B

19. B

20. C

21. D

22. D

23. A

24. D

25. A

26. C

27. D

28. C

29. D

30. B

Math Answer Key

1. A
1/3 X 3/4 = 3/12 = 1/4
To multiply fractions, multiply the numerator and denominator.

2. D
The question asks for approximate cost, so work with round numbers. The jacket costs $545.00 so we can round up to $550. 10% of $550 is 55. We can round down to $50, which is easier to work with. $550 - $50 is $500. The jacket will cost about $500.

The actual cost will be 10% X 545 = $54.50
545 – 54.50 = $490.50

3. D
3.14 + 2.73 = 5.87 and 5.87 + 23.7 = 29.57

4. C
To convert a decimal to a fraction, take the places of decimal as your denominator, here 2, so in 0.27, '7' is in the 100th place, so the fraction is 27/100 and 0.33 becomes 33/100.

Next estimate the answer quickly to eliminate obvious wrong choices. 27/100 is about 1/4 and 33/100 is 1/3. 1/3 is slightly larger than 1/4, and 1/4 + 1/4 is 1/2, so the answer will be slightly larger than 1/2.

Looking at the choices, choice A can be eliminated since 3/6 = 1/2. Choice D, 2/7 is less than 1/2 and be eliminated. The answer is going to be choice B or choice C.
Do the calculation, 0.27 + 0.33 = 0.60 and 0.60 = 60/100 = 3/5, Choice C is correct.

5. B
Spent 15% - 100% - 15% = 85%

6. C
This is an easy question, and shows how you can solve some questions without doing the calculations. The question is, 8 is what percent of 40. Take easy percentages for an approximate answer and see what you get.

10% is easy to calculate because you can drop the zero, or move the decimal point. 10% of 40 = 4, and 8 = 2 X 4, so, 8 must be 2 X 10% = 20%.

Here are the calculations which confirm the quick approximation.
8/40 = X/100 = 8 * 100 / 40X = 800/40 = X = 20

7. A
According to the graph, oil consumption peaked in 2011.

8. A
2 + a number divided by 7.
(2 + X) divided by 7.
(2 + X)/7

9. B
.4/100 * 36 = .4 * 36/100 = .144

10. A
5 mg/10/mg X 1 tab/1 = .5 tablets

11. B
Step 1: Set up the formula to calculate the dose to be given in mg as per weight of the child:-
Dose ordered X Weight in Kg = Dose to be given
Step 2: 20 mg X 12 kg = 240 mg
240 mg/80 mg X 1 tab/1 = 240/80 = 3 tablets

12. A
MCMXC is 1990. 1000 + (1000 − 100) + (100 − 10) = 1990

13. D
Indonesia is growing the fastest at about 30%.

14. B
$(4)(3^3) = (4)(27) = 108$

15. C
4 quarts = 1 gallon, 16 quarts = 16/4 = 4 gallons.

Conversion problems are easy to get confused. One way to think of them is which is larger - quarts or gallons? Gallons are larger, so if you are converting from quarts to gallons the number of gallons will be a smaller number. Keeping that in mind, you can do a 'common-sense' check on your answer.

16. B
0.45 kg = 1 pound, 1 kg. = 1/0.45 and 45 kg = 1/0.45 x 45 = 99.208, or 100 pounds.

17. C
Three plus a number times 7 equals 42. Let X be the number.
(3 + X) times 7 = 42
7(3 + X) = 42

18. B
Number of absent students = 83 – 72 = 11

Percentage of absent students is found by proportioning the number of absent students to total number of students in the class = 11•100/83 = 13.25

Checking the answers, we round 13.25 to the nearest whole number: 13%

19. C
To solve for x, first simplify the equation
5x + 2x + 14 = 14x – 7
7x + 14 = 4x -7
7x – 14x + 14 = -7
7x – 14x = -7 – 14
-7x = -21
x = -21/-7
x=3

20. C
5z + 5 = 3z +6 + 11
5z -3z + 5 =6 + 11
5z – 3z = 6 + 11 -5
2z = 17 – 5
2z = 12
z= 12/2
z= 6

21. D
Price increased by $5 ($25-$20). to calculate the percent increase:
5/20 = X/100
500 = 20X
X = 500/20
X = 25%

22. C
The ratio is 2 to 8, or 1:4.

23. D
2 glasses are broken for 43 customers so 1 glass breaks for every 43/2 customers served, therefore 10 glasses implies 43/2 x 10=215. She served 215 customers.

24. D
As the lawn is square shaped, the length of one side will be the square root of the area. √62,500 = 250 meters. So, the perimeter is found by 4 times the length of the side of the square:

250 * 4 = 1000 meters.

Since each meter costs $5.5, the total cost of the fence will be 1000 * 5.5 = $5,500.

25. B
5n + (19 – 2) = 67, 5n + 17 = 67, 5n = 67 -17, 5n = 50, n = 50/5 = 10

26. B

Day	Absent	Present	% Attendance
Monday	5	40	88.88%
Tuesday	9	36	80.00%
Wednesday	4	41	91.11%
Thursday	10	35	77.77%
Friday	6	39	86.66%

Sum of the percent attendance is 424.42. Divide by 5 for the average, 424.42/5 = 84.884. Round up to 85%.

27. B
The distribution is done in three different rates and amounts:

$6.4 per 20 kilograms to 15 shops ... 20•15 = 300 kilograms distributed

$3.4 per 10 kilograms to 12 shops ... 10•12 = 120 kilograms distributed

550 - (300 + 120) = 550 - 420 = 130 kilograms left. This amount is distributed by 5 kilogram portions. So, this means that there are 130/5 = 26 shops.

$1.8 per 130 kilograms.

We need to find the amount he earned overall these distributions.

$6.4 per 20 kilograms : 6.4•15 = $96 for 300 kilograms

$3.4 per 10 kilograms : 3.4•12 = $40.8 for 120 kilograms

$1.8 per 5 kilograms : 1.8•26 = $46.8 for 130 kilograms

So, he earned 96 + 40.8 + 46.8 = $ 183.6

The total distribution cost is given as $10

The profit is found by: Money earned - money spent ... It is important to remember that he bought 550 kilograms of potatoes for $165 at the beginning:

Profit = 183.6 - 10 - 165 = $8.6

28. B
We check the fractions taking place in the question. We see that there is a "half" (that is 1/2) and 3/7. So, we multiply the denominators of these fractions to decide how to name the total money. We say that Mr. Johnson has 14x at the beginning; he gives half of this, meaning 7x, to his family. $250 to his landlord. He has 3/7 of his money left. 3/7 of 14x is equal to:

14x•(3/7) = 6x

So,

Spent money is: 7x + 250

Unspent money is: 6x

Total money is: 14x

We write an equation: total money = spent money + unspent money

14x = 7x + 250 + 6x

14x - 7x - 6x = 250

x = 250

We are asked to find the total money that is 14x:

14x = 14•250 = $3500

29. A
The probability that the 1st ball drawn is red = 4/11
The probability that the 2nd ball drawn is green = 5/10
The combined probability will then be 4/11 X 5/10 = 20/110 = 2/11

30. D

First calculate total square feet, which is 15•24 = 360 ft2. Next, convert this vaue to square yards, (1 yards2 = 9 ft2) which is 360/9 = 40 yards2. At $0.50 per square yard, the total cost is 40•0.50 = $20.

Section III – Nonverbal

1. D

The relation is the same figure rotated.

2. D

The shaded area is divided in half in the second figure.

3. D

The relation is the same figure rotated to the right.

4. B

The relation is the number of dots is one-half the number of sides.

5. C

The pattern is the same figure with a dot inside.

6. A

The relation is the same figure smaller, plus another figure with one more side.

7. B

The relation is the bottom half of the figure.

8. C

The relation is the right half of the first object.

9. B

The relation is the right half of the first object.

10. D

Each time the * and + alternate, either singly or doubles.

11. D

This is a place relationship. Acting is done in a theater in the same way gambling is done in a casino.

12. C

Pork is the meat of a pig in the same way beef is the meat of a cow.

13. A

This is a classification relationship. The first is the class which the second belongs.

14. C

Slumber is a synonym for sleep and bog is a synonym for swamp.

15. B

The first is the study of the second. Zoology is the study of animals in the same way botany is the study of plants.

16. B

This is a type relationship. A child is a young human just as a kitten is a young cat.

17. B

This is a composition relationship. A candle is made of wax and a bowl is made of clay.

18. C

A kite is not a type of plane.

19. D

This is a relationship of words question. All the choices are synonyms of count, except figure.

20. B

This is a capital small letter relationship. All choices start with a capital letter.

21. D

BD is not a sequence of consecutive letters.

22. C

This is a repetition pattern. All the choices repeat a 2-letter sequence.

23. B

123 are consecutive, the others are obtained by adding 2.

24. C

ACF is not a sequence of consecutive letters.

25. C

Capital small letter relationship. All choices have the middle two letters capitalized except c.

26. A

This is a vowel and consonant relationship. All the choices are only consonants, except Choice A.

27. C

This is a vowel and consonant relationship. All the choices have 2 vowels at the end.

28. B

246 is not a sequence of consecutive numbers.

29. D

This is a vowel and consonant relationship. All the choices have one vowel in the middle position.

30. B

This is a word meaning relationship. Talk is not a synonym for any of the choices.

Part II – Spelling

1. C
2. D
3. C
4. A
5. C
6. C
7. A
8. B
9. A
10. B
11. C
12. A
13. D
14. C
15. B
16. C
17. C
18. A
19. C
20. B
21. B

22. D
23. B
24. C
25. A
26. B
27. C
28. D
29. A
30. B

Section III – Reading Comprehension

1. B
We can infer from this passage that sickness from an infectious disease can be easily transmitted from one person to another.

From the passage, "Infectious pathologies are also called communicable diseases or transmissible diseases, due to their potential of transmission from one person or species to another by a replicating agent (as opposed to a toxin)."

2. A
Two other names for infectious pathologies are communicable diseases and transmissible diseases.

From the passage, "Infectious pathologies are also called communicable diseases or transmissible diseases, due to their potential of transmission from one person or species to another by a replicating agent (as opposed to a toxin)."

3. C
Infectivity describes the ability of an organism to enter, survive and multiply in the host. This is taken directly from the passage, and is a definition type question.

Definition type questions can be answered quickly and easily by scanning the passage for the word you are asked to define.

"Infectivity" is an unusual word, so it is quick and easy to scan the passage looking for this word.

4. B
We know an infection is not synonymous with an infectious disease because an infection may not cause important clinical symptoms or impair host function.

5. C
We can infer from the passage that, a virus is too small to be seen with the naked eye. Clearly, if they are too small to be seen with a microscope, then they are too

small to be seen with the naked eye.

6. D
Viruses infect all types of organisms. This is taken directly from the passage, "Viruses infect all types of organisms, from animals and plants to bacteria and single-celled organisms."

7. C
The passage does not say exactly how many parts prions and viroids consist of. It does say, "Unlike prions and viroids, viruses consist of two or three parts ..." so we can infer they consist of either less than two or more than three parts.

8. B
A common virus spread by coughing and sneezing is Influenza.

9. C
The cumulus stage of a thunderstorm is the beginning of the thunderstorm.

This is taken directly from the passage, "The first stage of a thunderstorm is the cumulus, or developing stage."

10. D
The passage lists four ways that air is heated. One way is, heat created by water vapor condensing into liquid.

11. A
The sequence of events can be taken from these sentences:

As the moisture carried by the [1] air currents rises, it rapidly cools into liquid drops of water, which appear as cumulus clouds. As the water vapor condenses into liquid, it [2] releases heat, which warms the air. This in turn causes the air to become less dense than the surrounding dry air and [3] rise farther.

12. C
The purpose of this text is to explain when meteorologists consider a thunderstorm severe.

The main idea is the first sentence, "The United States National Weather Service classifies thunderstorms as severe when they reach a predetermined level." After the first sentence, the passage explains and elaborates on this idea. Everything is this passage is related to this idea, and there are no other major ideas in this passage that are central to the whole passage.

13. A
From this passage, we can infer that different areas and countries have different criteria for determining a severe storm.

From the passage we can see that most of the US has a criteria of, winds over 50 knots (58 mph or 93 km/h), and hail ¾ inch (2 cm). For the Central US, hail must be 1 inch (2.5 cm) in diameter. In Canada, winds must be 90 km/h or greater, hail 2 centimeters in diameter or greater, and rainfall more than 50 millimeters in 1 hour, or 75 millimeters in 3 hours.

Choice D is incorrect because the Canadian system is the same for hail, 2 centimeters in diameter.

14. C

With hail above the minimum size of 2.5 cm. diameter, the Central Region of the United States National Weather Service would issue a severe thunderstorm warning.

15. C

You would find information about natural selection and adaptation in the ecology section which begins on page 110.

16. D

Clouds in space are made of different materials attracted by gravity. Clouds on Earth are made of water droplets or ice crystals.

Choice D is the best answer. Notice also that Choice D is the most specific.

17. C

The main idea is the first sentence of the passage; a cloud is a visible mass of droplets or frozen crystals floating in the atmosphere above the surface of the Earth or other planetary body.

The main idea is very often the first sentence of the paragraph.

18. C

Nephology, which is the study of cloud physics.

19. C

This question asks about the process, and gives choices that can be confirmed or eliminated easily.

From the passage, "Dense, deep clouds reflect most light, so they appear white, at least from the top. Cloud droplets scatter light very efficiently, so the farther into a cloud light travels, the weaker it gets. This accounts for the gray or dark appearance at the base of large clouds."

We can eliminate choice A, since water droplets inside the cloud do not reflect light is false.

We can eliminate choice B, since, water droplets outside the cloud reflect light, it appears dark, is false.

Choice C is correct.

20. A
We know that an annex is like an attic because the text states the annex was above Otto Frank's building.

Option B is incorrect because an office building doesn't have bedrooms. Option C is incorrect because a basement would be below the office building. Option D is incorrect because there would not be a kitchen in an office building.

21. B
The diary has been published in 55 languages so people all over the world can learn about Anne. That is why the passage says it has been continuously in print.

Option A is incorrect because it is too vague. Option C is incorrect because it was published after Anne died and she did not write in all three languages. Option D is incorrect because the passage does not give us any information about what languages Otto Frank spoke.

22. C
Use the process of elimination to figure this out.

Option A cannot be the correct answer because otherwise the passage would have simply said that Anne and Margot both died of starvation. Options B and D cannot be correct because if the Germans had done something specifically to murder Anne, the passage would have stated that directly. By the process of elimination, Option C has to be the correct answer.

23. D
We can figure this out using context clues. The paragraph is talking about Anne's diary and so, outlet in this instance is a place where Anne can pour her feelings.

Option A is incorrect answer. That is the literal meaning of the word outlet and the passage is using the figurative meaning. Option B is incorrect because that is the secondary literal meaning of the word outlet, as in an outlet mall. Again, we are looking for figurative meaning. Option C is incorrect because there are no clues in the text to support that answer.

24. B
Reading the document posted to the Human Resources website is optional.

25. B
The document is recommended changes and have not be implemented yet.

26. A

Navy SEALs are the maritime component of the United States Special Operations Command (USSOCOM).

27. C

Working underwater separates SEALs from other military units. This is taken directly from the passage.

28. D

SEALs also belong to the Navy and the Coast Guard.

29. A

The CIA also participated. From the passage, the raid was conducted by a "team of 40 *CIA-led* Navy SEALs."

30. C

According to the blood pressure gauge, the patient's pulse is 62 beats per minute.

31. B

When someone is avid about something that means they are highly interested in the subject. The context clues are dull and boring, because they define the opposite of avid.

32. A

The author is using a simile to compare the books to medicine. Medicine is what you take when you want to feel better. They are suggesting that if a person wants to feel good, they should read Dr. Seuss' books.

Option B is incorrect because there is no mention of a doctor's office. Option C is incorrect because it is using the literal meaning of medicine and the author is using medicine in a figurative way. Option D is incorrect because it makes no sense. We know not to eat books.

33. D

The publisher is described as intelligent because he knew to get in touch with a famous author to develop a book that children would be interested in reading.

Option A is incorrect because we can assume that all book publishers must know how to read. Option B is incorrect because it says in the article that more than one publisher was concerned about whether or not children liked to read. Option D is incorrect because there is no mention in the article about how well The Cat in the Hat sold when it was first published.

34. A

The Save the Children's fund has raised $12,000 out of $20,000, or 12/20. Simplifying, 12/20 = 3/5

35. B
The Save the Children's fund has raised $12,000 out of $16,000, or 12/16. Simplifying, 12/16 = 3/4

Section IV – Basic Science

1. A
Phenotype refers to observed properties of an organism and genotype refers to the genes of an organism.

2. A
A solution with a pH value of greater than 7 is a base.

3. A
Eukaryotic and prokaryotic cells are both organelles.

4. C
Homologous is being inherited by the organisms' common ancestors. An example would be feathers and hair—both of which were structures that shared a common ancestral trait.

5. C
The manner in which instructions for building proteins, the basic structural molecules of living material are written in the DNA is a genetic code.

6. C
A gene is a unit of inherited material, encoded by a strand of DNA and transcribed by RNA.

7. D
All of these statements are correct.

  a. During meiosis, the number of chromosomes in the cell are halved.

  b. Meiosis only occurs in eukaryotic cells.

  c. Meiosis is the part of the life cycle that involves sexual reproduction.

8. A Carrying capacity
An area's carrying capacity is the maximum number of animals of a given species that area can support during the harshest part of the year.

9. B
Diverticulitis is a pouch in the large intestine becomes inflamed.

10. A
Detection of pathogens can be complicated because they evolve so quickly.

11. A
Photosynthesis is the process by which plants and other photoautotrophs generate carbohydrates and oxygen from carbon dioxide, water, and light energy in chloroplasts.

12. C
Mutations in DNA sequences usually occur spontaneously is false.

Note: Mutations result when the DNA polymerase makes a mistake, which happens about once every 100,000,000 bases. Actually, the number of mistakes that remain incorporated into the DNA is even lower than this because cells contain special DNA repair proteins that fix many of the mistakes in the DNA that are caused by mutagens. The repair proteins see which nucleotides are paired incorrectly, and then change the wrong base to the right one. [14]

13. A
Starting with the weakest, the fundamental forces of nature in order of strength are, Gravity, Weak nuclear force, Electromagnetic force, Strong nuclear force.

Note: Although gravitational force is the weakest of the four, it acts over great distances. Electromagnetic force is of order 10^{39} times stronger than gravity.

14. A
Precision, which refers to the repeatability of measurement, does not require knowledge of the correct or true value.

15. A
Artificial selection is a process where desirable traits are systematically bred.

16. C
Condensation is not an example of vaporization. Boiling and evaporation are both examples of vaporization. Condensation is the process by which matter transitions from a gas to a liquid.

17. B
A periodic table is a tabular display of the chemical elements, organized on the basis of their atomic numbers, electron configurations, and recurring chemical properties.

18. A
In terms of the scientific method, the term observation refers to the act of noticing or perceiving something and/or recording a fact or occurrence.

19. B
Kinetic energy is the energy of a body that results from motion while potential energy is the energy possessed by an object by virtue of its position or state, e.g., as in a compressed spring.

20. A
A life cycle is the sequence of developmental stages through which members of a given species must pass.

21. A
The cell membrane is a biological membrane that separates the interior of all cells from the outside environment. The cell membrane is selectively permeable to ions and organic molecules and controls the movement of substances in and out of cells [15]

22. D
Relative position is not a taxonomic rank. Ranks include Domain, Kingdom, Phylum, Class, Order, Family, Genus, and Species.

23. D
The scientific term experiment refers to a practical test designed with the intention that its results be relevant to a particular theory or set of theories.

24. B
Substances that deactivate catalysts are called catalytic poisons.

25. B
Kinetic energy is the energy an object possesses due to its motion.

26. C
The interval of confidence around the measured value such that the measured value is certain not to lie outside this stated interval refers to the **uncertainty** of that value.

27. D
Arteries carry oxygenated blood away from the heart, veins return oxygen-depleted blood to the heart, and capillaries are thin-walled blood vessels in which gas/ nutrient/ waste exchange occurs.

Note: An easy way to remember the difference between an artery and a vein is that Arteries carry Away from the heart.

28. B
The thoracic diaphragm, or simply the diaphragm, is a sheet of internal skeletal muscle that extends across the bottom of the rib cage. The diaphragm separates the thoracic cavity (heart, lungs & ribs) from the abdominal cavity and performs an important function in respiration. [16]

29. D
Scientific classification. The two phrases are interchangeable, although the former seems to more accurately reflect the purpose of classification: to categorize biological units.

30. C
A recessive gene is not expressed as a trait unless inherited by both parents.

31. D
A scientific model is an approximation or simulation of a real system that omits all but the most essential variables of the system.

32. A
Neutrons are necessary within an atomic nucleus as they bind with protons via the nuclear force.

33. C
The following statement is false - Most enzymes are inorganic.

34. C
Acids are compounds that contain hydrogen and can dissolve in water to release hydrogen ions into solution.

35. A
Genes determine individual hereditary characteristics

36. A
The groups into which organisms are classified are called taxa and include, **in order of size**, Genus, Kingdom, Phylum/division, Class, Order, and Family Species.

37. D
Digestion begins in the mouth.

38. A
The main components of the circulatory system are the heart, veins and blood

vessels.

39. D
An example of a pathogen that the immune system detects is a virus.

40. A
Chemical bonds are attractions between atoms that form chemical substances containing two or more atoms.

41. B
Cleansing food of impurities is not an example of a function of the stomach in digestion.

42. D
The exchange of oxygen for carbon dioxide takes place in the alveolar area of the lungs.

43. C
In chemistry, the number of protons in the nucleus of an atom is known as the atomic number, which determines the chemical element to which the atom belongs.

44. C
Natural selection is a process where biological traits become more or less common in a population

45. A
Females have two X chromosomes and males have one X chromosome and one Y chromosome.

46. A
The immune system fight off disease by identifying and killing tumor cells and pathogens.

47. A
Water has two hydrogen atoms covalently bonded to one oxygen atom

48. C
Choice C (Atomic theory explains temperature as the momentum of atoms.) is incorrect because atomic theory explains temperature as the motion of atoms (faster = hotter), not the momentum. The momentum of atoms explains the outward pressure that they exert. [17]

49. D
Cardiac dysrhythmia (also known as arrhythmia and irregular heartbeat) is a term for any of a large and heterogeneous group of conditions in which there is abnormal electrical activity in the heart. The heart beat may be too fast or too slow, and may be regular or irregular. [18]

50. A
Eating a healthy diet is the best way to avoid most digestive diseases.

51. C
An important side-benefit of the respiratory system is the air being expelled from the mouth allows for speaking.

52. A
Emphysema is a long-term, progressive disease of the lungs that primarily causes shortness of breath. In people with emphysema, the tissues necessary to support the physical shape and function of the lungs are destroyed. It is included in a group of diseases called chronic obstructive pulmonary disease or COPD (pulmonary refers to the lungs). [19]

53. B
Inflammation is an example of an early response by the immune system to infection.

54. B
White blood cells are an important weapon in the fight against infection?

55. A
The complementary bases found in DNA are adenine and thymine or cytosine and guanine.

56. A
The term genome may be applied to the genetic information carried by an individual or to the range of genes found in a given species. The human genome is composed of 75,000 genes.

57. B
Taxonomy is a classification of organisms into different categories based on their physical characteristics and presumed natural relationship.

58. A
The order of the hierarchy of levels in the biological classification of organisms is: Kingdom, phylum, class, order, family, genus, and species.

59. A
A salt is any compound produced by a chemical reaction between a base and an acid.

60. A
A food web is a graphical description of feeding relationships among species in an ecological community.

Note: A food web differs from a food chain in that the latter shows only a portion of the food web involving a simple, linear series of species (e.g., predator, herbivore, plant) connected by feeding links. A food web aims to depict a more complete picture of the feeding relationships, and can be considered a bundle of many interconnected food chains occurring within the community.

Practice Test 2

Part 1 - Academic Aptitude

Verbal Sub-test – Vocabulary
Questions: 30
Time: 30 Minutes

Mathematics Sub-test
Questions: 30
Time: 30 Minutes

Nonverbal Sub-test
Questions: 30
Time: 30 Minutes

Part II – Spelling
Questions: 30
Time: 30 Minutes

Part III – Reading Comprehension
Questions: 35
Time: 35 Minutes

Part VI – Basic Science
Questions: 60
Time: 60 minutes

The practice test portion presents questions that are representative of the type of question you should expect to find on the PSB. However, they are not intended to match exactly what is on the PSB. Don't worry though! If you can answer these questions, you will have not trouble with the PSB.

For the best results, take this Practice Test as if it were the real exam. Set aside time when you will not be disturbed, and a location that is quiet and free of distractions. Read the instructions carefully, read each question carefully, and answer to the best of your ability.

Use the bubble answer sheets provided. When you have completed the Practice Test, check your answer against the Answer Key and read the explanation provided.

Answer Sheet – Part 1 – Vocabulary Sub-test

1. Ⓐ Ⓑ Ⓒ Ⓓ   11. Ⓐ Ⓑ Ⓒ Ⓓ   21. Ⓐ Ⓑ Ⓒ Ⓓ

2. Ⓐ Ⓑ Ⓒ Ⓓ   12. Ⓐ Ⓑ Ⓒ Ⓓ   22. Ⓐ Ⓑ Ⓒ Ⓓ

3. Ⓐ Ⓑ Ⓒ Ⓓ   13. Ⓐ Ⓑ Ⓒ Ⓓ   23. Ⓐ Ⓑ Ⓒ Ⓓ

4. Ⓐ Ⓑ Ⓒ Ⓓ   14. Ⓐ Ⓑ Ⓒ Ⓓ   24. Ⓐ Ⓑ Ⓒ Ⓓ

5. Ⓐ Ⓑ Ⓒ Ⓓ   15. Ⓐ Ⓑ Ⓒ Ⓓ   25. Ⓐ Ⓑ Ⓒ Ⓓ

6. Ⓐ Ⓑ Ⓒ Ⓓ   16. Ⓐ Ⓑ Ⓒ Ⓓ   26. Ⓐ Ⓑ Ⓒ Ⓓ

7. Ⓐ Ⓑ Ⓒ Ⓓ   17. Ⓐ Ⓑ Ⓒ Ⓓ   27. Ⓐ Ⓑ Ⓒ Ⓓ

8. Ⓐ Ⓑ Ⓒ Ⓓ   18. Ⓐ Ⓑ Ⓒ Ⓓ   28. Ⓐ Ⓑ Ⓒ Ⓓ

9. Ⓐ Ⓑ Ⓒ Ⓓ   19. Ⓐ Ⓑ Ⓒ Ⓓ   29. Ⓐ Ⓑ Ⓒ Ⓓ

10. Ⓐ Ⓑ Ⓒ Ⓓ   20. Ⓐ Ⓑ Ⓒ Ⓓ   30. Ⓐ Ⓑ Ⓒ Ⓓ

Answer Sheet – Part I – Mathematics Sub-test

1. (A) (B) (C) (D)   11. (A) (B) (C) (D)   21. (A) (B) (C) (D)

2. (A) (B) (C) (D)   12. (A) (B) (C) (D)   22. (A) (B) (C) (D)

3. (A) (B) (C) (D)   13. (A) (B) (C) (D)   23. (A) (B) (C) (D)

4. (A) (B) (C) (D)   14. (A) (B) (C) (D)   24. (A) (B) (C) (D)

5. (A) (B) (C) (D)   15. (A) (B) (C) (D)   25. (A) (B) (C) (D)

6. (A) (B) (C) (D)   16. (A) (B) (C) (D)   26. (A) (B) (C) (D)

7. (A) (B) (C) (D)   17. (A) (B) (C) (D)   27. (A) (B) (C) (D)

8. (A) (B) (C) (D)   18. (A) (B) (C) (D)   28. (A) (B) (C) (D)

9. (A) (B) (C) (D)   19. (A) (B) (C) (D)   29. (A) (B) (C) (D)

10. (A) (B) (C) (D)   20. (A) (B) (C) (D)   30. (A) (B) (C) (D)

Answer Sheet – Part I – Nonverbal Sub-test

1. (A) (B) (C) (D)   11. (A) (B) (C) (D)   21. (A) (B) (C) (D)

2. (A) (B) (C) (D)   12. (A) (B) (C) (D)   22. (A) (B) (C) (D)

3. (A) (B) (C) (D)   13. (A) (B) (C) (D)   23. (A) (B) (C) (D)

4. (A) (B) (C) (D)   14. (A) (B) (C) (D)   24. (A) (B) (C) (D)

5. (A) (B) (C) (D)   15. (A) (B) (C) (D)   25. (A) (B) (C) (D)

6. (A) (B) (C) (D)   16. (A) (B) (C) (D)   26. (A) (B) (C) (D)

7. (A) (B) (C) (D)   17. (A) (B) (C) (D)   27. (A) (B) (C) (D)

8. (A) (B) (C) (D)   18. (A) (B) (C) (D)   28. (A) (B) (C) (D)

9. (A) (B) (C) (D)   19. (A) (B) (C) (D)   29. (A) (B) (C) (D)

10. (A) (B) (C) (D)   20. (A) (B) (C) (D)   30. (A) (B) (C) (D)

Answer Sheet - Part II – Spelling

1. (A) (B) (C) (D)   11. (A) (B) (C) (D)   21. (A) (B) (C) (D)

2. (A) (B) (C) (D)   12. (A) (B) (C) (D)   22. (A) (B) (C) (D)

3. (A) (B) (C) (D)   13. (A) (B) (C) (D)   23. (A) (B) (C) (D)

4. (A) (B) (C) (D)   14. (A) (B) (C) (D)   24. (A) (B) (C) (D)

5. (A) (B) (C) (D)   15. (A) (B) (C) (D)   25. (A) (B) (C) (D)

6. (A) (B) (C) (D)   16. (A) (B) (C) (D)   26. (A) (B) (C) (D)

7. (A) (B) (C) (D)   17. (A) (B) (C) (D)   27. (A) (B) (C) (D)

8. (A) (B) (C) (D)   18. (A) (B) (C) (D)   28. (A) (B) (C) (D)

9. (A) (B) (C) (D)   19. (A) (B) (C) (D)   29. (A) (B) (C) (D)

10. (A) (B) (C) (D)   20. (A) (B) (C) (D)   30. (A) (B) (C) (D)

Answer Sheet – Part III – Reading Comprehension

1. Ⓐ Ⓑ Ⓒ Ⓓ   11. Ⓐ Ⓑ Ⓒ Ⓓ   21. Ⓐ Ⓑ Ⓒ Ⓓ   31. Ⓐ Ⓑ Ⓒ Ⓓ

2. Ⓐ Ⓑ Ⓒ Ⓓ   12. Ⓐ Ⓑ Ⓒ Ⓓ   22. Ⓐ Ⓑ Ⓒ Ⓓ   32. Ⓐ Ⓑ Ⓒ Ⓓ

3. Ⓐ Ⓑ Ⓒ Ⓓ   13. Ⓐ Ⓑ Ⓒ Ⓓ   23. Ⓐ Ⓑ Ⓒ Ⓓ   33. Ⓐ Ⓑ Ⓒ Ⓓ

4. Ⓐ Ⓑ Ⓒ Ⓓ   14. Ⓐ Ⓑ Ⓒ Ⓓ   24. Ⓐ Ⓑ Ⓒ Ⓓ   34. Ⓐ Ⓑ Ⓒ Ⓓ

5. Ⓐ Ⓑ Ⓒ Ⓓ   15. Ⓐ Ⓑ Ⓒ Ⓓ   25. Ⓐ Ⓑ Ⓒ Ⓓ   35. Ⓐ Ⓑ Ⓒ Ⓓ

6. Ⓐ Ⓑ Ⓒ Ⓓ   16. Ⓐ Ⓑ Ⓒ Ⓓ   26. Ⓐ Ⓑ Ⓒ Ⓓ

7. Ⓐ Ⓑ Ⓒ Ⓓ   17. Ⓐ Ⓑ Ⓒ Ⓓ   27. Ⓐ Ⓑ Ⓒ Ⓓ

8. Ⓐ Ⓑ Ⓒ Ⓓ   18. Ⓐ Ⓑ Ⓒ Ⓓ   28. Ⓐ Ⓑ Ⓒ Ⓓ

9. Ⓐ Ⓑ Ⓒ Ⓓ   19. Ⓐ Ⓑ Ⓒ Ⓓ   29. Ⓐ Ⓑ Ⓒ Ⓓ

10. Ⓐ Ⓑ Ⓒ Ⓓ   20. Ⓐ Ⓑ Ⓒ Ⓓ   30. Ⓐ Ⓑ Ⓒ Ⓓ

Answer Sheet – Part IV - Natural Sciences

1. (A) (B) (C) (D)	21. (A) (B) (C) (D)	41. (A) (B) (C) (D)	61. (A) (B) (C) (D)
2. (A) (B) (C) (D)	22. (A) (B) (C) (D)	42. (A) (B) (C) (D)	62. (A) (B) (C) (D)
3. (A) (B) (C) (D)	23. (A) (B) (C) (D)	43. (A) (B) (C) (D)	63. (A) (B) (C) (D)
4. (A) (B) (C) (D)	24. (A) (B) (C) (D)	44. (A) (B) (C) (D)	64. (A) (B) (C) (D)
5. (A) (B) (C) (D)	25. (A) (B) (C) (D)	45. (A) (B) (C) (D)	65. (A) (B) (C) (D)
6. (A) (B) (C) (D)	26. (A) (B) (C) (D)	46. (A) (B) (C) (D)	66. (A) (B) (C) (D)
7. (A) (B) (C) (D)	27. (A) (B) (C) (D)	47. (A) (B) (C) (D)	67. (A) (B) (C) (D)
8. (A) (B) (C) (D)	28. (A) (B) (C) (D)	48. (A) (B) (C) (D)	68. (A) (B) (C) (D)
9. (A) (B) (C) (D)	29. (A) (B) (C) (D)	49. (A) (B) (C) (D)	69. (A) (B) (C) (D)
10. (A) (B) (C) (D)	30. (A) (B) (C) (D)	50. (A) (B) (C) (D)	70. (A) (B) (C) (D)
11. (A) (B) (C) (D)	31. (A) (B) (C) (D)	51. (A) (B) (C) (D)	71. (A) (B) (C) (D)
12. (A) (B) (C) (D)	32. (A) (B) (C) (D)	52. (A) (B) (C) (D)	72. (A) (B) (C) (D)
13. (A) (B) (C) (D)	33. (A) (B) (C) (D)	53. (A) (B) (C) (D)	73. (A) (B) (C) (D)
14. (A) (B) (C) (D)	34. (A) (B) (C) (D)	54. (A) (B) (C) (D)	74. (A) (B) (C) (D)
15. (A) (B) (C) (D)	35. (A) (B) (C) (D)	55. (A) (B) (C) (D)	75. (A) (B) (C) (D)
16. (A) (B) (C) (D)	36. (A) (B) (C) (D)	56. (A) (B) (C) (D)	76. (A) (B) (C) (D)
17. (A) (B) (C) (D)	37. (A) (B) (C) (D)	57. (A) (B) (C) (D)	77. (A) (B) (C) (D)
18. (A) (B) (C) (D)	38. (A) (B) (C) (D)	58. (A) (B) (C) (D)	78. (A) (B) (C) (D)
19. (A) (B) (C) (D)	39. (A) (B) (C) (D)	59. (A) (B) (C) (D)	79. (A) (B) (C) (D)
20. (A) (B) (C) (D)	40. (A) (B) (C) (D)	60. (A) (B) (C) (D)	80. (A) (B) (C) (D)

Part 1 – Academic Aptitude - Vocabulary

1. a. Exigent b. Accurate c. Precise d. Undemanding

2. a. Inimical b. Amicable c. Friendly d. Sociable

3. a. Grapple b. Seize c. Prebend d. Unleash

4. a. Pervious b. Receptive c. Timorous d. Porous

5. a. Exorbitant b. Expensive c. Unconscionable d. Moderate

6. a. Unctuous b. Reprehensible c. Deplorable d. Vicious

7. a. Persuasive b. Admonitory c. Cautionary d. Exemplary

8. a. Talk b. Ponder c. Speak d. Pontificate

9. a. Address b. Speak c. Harangue d. Query

10. a. Adjourn b. Convoke c. Convene d. Summon

11. a. Decode b. Conform c. Decrypt d. Decipher

12. a. Discharge b. Exonerate c. Convict d. Exculpate

13. a. Elucidate b. Obfuscate c. Explain d. Explicate

14. a. Ardent b. Fervent c. Passionless d. Torrid

15. a. Taciturn b. Garrulous c. Loquacious d. Talkative

16. a. Intrepid b. Fearless c. Craven d. Brave

17. a. Jocular b. Amusing c. Uproarious d. Sober

18. a. Judicious b. Prudent c. Irrational d. Cautious

19. a. Lacerate b. Wound c. Rip d. Inculcate

20. a. Obligatory b. Elective c. Indispensable d. Prerequisite

21. a. Obsolete b. Objectionable c. Obnoxious d. Annoying

22. a. Rankle b. Grate c. Annoy d. Ingratiate

23. a. Verdure b. Greenness c. Freshness d. Expansive

24. a. Enthusiast b. Extremist c. Champion d. Zealot

25. a. Lithe b. Flexible c. Pliant d. Artificial

26. a. Pudgy b. Plump c. Overdone d. Fat

27. a. Aggravate b. Mollify c. Soothe d. Allay

28. a. Vex b. Assist c. Agitate d. Exasperate

29. a. Oblivious b. Abeyance c. Conscious d. Insensible

30. a. Abominate   b. Abhor   c. Cherish   d. Loathe

Mathematics

1. Richard gives 's' amount of salary to each of his 'n' employees weekly. If he has 'x' amount of money then how many days he can employ these 'n' employees.

    a. sx/7n

    b. 7x/nx

    c. nx/7s

    d. 7x/ns

2. Translate the following into an equation: Five greater than 3 times a number.

    a. 3X + 5

    b. 5X + 3

    c. (5 + 3)X

    d. 5(3 + X)

3. What number is MMXIII?

    a. 2010

    b. 1990

    c. 2013

    d. 2012

4. It is known that $x^2+4x=5$. Then x can be

    a. 0

    b. -5

    c. 1

    d. Either (b) or (c)

5. Write 765.3682 to the nearest 1000th.

    a. 765.368

    b. 765.361

    c. 765.369

    d. 765.378

6. If Lynn can type a page in p minutes, what portion of the page can she do in 5 minutes?

    a. 5/p

    b. p - 5

    c. p + 5

    d. p/5

7. If Sally can paint a house in 4 hours, and John can paint the same house in 6 hours, how long will it take for both of them to paint the house together?

    a. 2 hours and 24 minutes

    b. 3 hours and 12 minutes

    c. 3 hours and 44 minutes

    d. 4 hours and 10 minutes

8. Employees of a discount appliance store receive an additional 20% off the lowest price on any item. If an employee purchases a dishwasher during a 15% off sale, how much will he pay if the dishwasher originally cost $450?

    a. $280.90

    b. $287

    c. $292.50

    d. $306

9. The sale price of a car is $12,590, which is 20% off the original price. What is the original price?

    a. $14,310.40

    b. $14,990.90

    c. $15,108.00

    d. $15,737.50

10. Express 25% as a fraction.

    a. 1/4

    b. 7/40

    c. 6/25

    d. 8/28

11. Express 125% as a decimal.

    a. .125

    b. 12.5

    c. 1.25

    d. 125

12. Express 24/56 as a reduced common fraction.

    a. 4/9

    b. 4/11

    c. 3/7

    d. 3/8

13. Express 71/1000 as a decimal.

    a. .71

    b. .0071

    c. .071

    d. 7.1

14. What number is in the ten thousandths place in 1.7389?

    a. 1

    b. 8

    c. 9

    d. 3

15. Simplify 6 3/5 – 4 4/5

    a. 2 4/5

    b. 2 3/5

    c. 2 9/5

    d. 1 1/5

16. The physician ordered 100 mg Ibuprofen/kg of body weight; on hand is 230 mg/tablet. The child weighs 50 lb. How many tablets will you give?

    a. 10 tablets

    b. 5 tablets

    c. 1 tablet

    d. 12 tablets

17. In a local election at polling station A, 945 voters cast their vote out of 1270 registered voters. At polling station B, 860 cast their vote out of 1050 registered voters and at station C, 1210 cast their vote out of 1440 registered voters. What is the total turnout including all three polling stations?

    a. 70%

    b. 74%

    c. 76%

    d. 80%

18. The physician ordered 600 mg ibuprofen. The office stocks 200 mg tablets. How many tablets will you give?

    a. 3.5 tablets

    b. 2 tablets

    c. 5 tablets

    d. 3 tablets

19. The manager of a weaving factory estimates that if 10 machines run on 100% efficiency for 8 hours, they will produce 1450 meters of cloth. However, due to some technical problems, 4 machines run of 95% efficiency and the remaining 6 at 90% efficiency. How many meters of cloth can these machines will produce in 8 hours?

    a. 1479 meters

    b. 1310 meters

    c. 1334 meters

    d. 1285 meters

20. Convert 60 feet to inches.

    a. 700 inches

    b. 600 inches

    c. 720 inches

    d. 1,800 inches

21. A box contains 7 black pencils and 28 blue ones. What is the ratio between the black and blue pens?

    a. 1:4

    b. 2:7

    c. 1:8

    d. 1:9

22. Convert 100 millimeters to centimeters.

    a. 10 centimeters

    b. 1,000 centimeters

    c. 1100 centimeters

    d. 50 centimeters

23. Convert 3 gallons to quarts.

    a. 15 quarts

    b. 6 quarts

    c. 12 quarts

    d. 32 quarts

24. A map uses a scale of 1:2,000 How much distance on the ground is 5.2 inches on the map if the scale is in inches?

     a. 100,400

     b. 10, 500

     c. 10,400

     d. 10,440

25. 0.05 ml. =

     a. 50 liters

     b. 0.00005 liters

     c. 5 liters

     d. 0.0005 liters

26. X% of 120 = 30. Solve for X.

     a. 15

     b. 12

     c. 4

     d. 25

27. Smith and Simon are playing a card game. Smith will win if a card drawn from a deck of 52 is either 7 or a diamond, and Simon will win if the drawn card is an even number. Which statement is more likely to be correct?

     a. Smith will win more games.

     b. Simon will win more games.

     c. They have same winning probability.

     d. A decision cannot be made from the provided data.

28. Convert .45 meters to centimeters

     a. 45

     b. 450

     c. 4.5

     d. .45

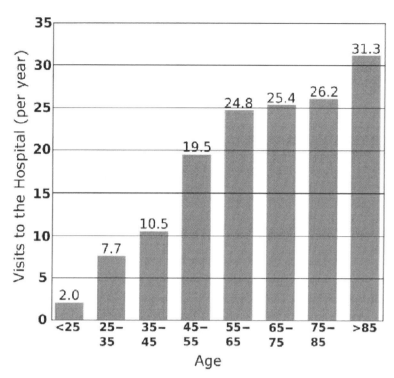

29. Consider the graph above.

How many hospital visits per year does a person aged 85 or more make?

   a. 26.2

   b. 31.3

   c. More than 31.3

   d. A decision cannot be made from this graph.

30. Based on this graph, how many visits per year do you expect a person that is 95 or older to make?

   a. More than 31.3

   b. Less than 31.3

   c. 31.3

   d. A decision cannot be made from this graph.

Nonverbal

1.

⬠ is to ⬠

△ is to ?

a. ▽   b. ◁

c. ▷   d. ⬭

2.

△ is to ▷

▯ is to ?

a. ▷   b. □

c. ⬠   d. ⬭

3.

▭ is to △

△ is to ?

a. △   b. □

c. ⬠   d. ▯

4.

□ is to ▭

△ is to ?

a. △   b. △

c. ⬠   d. ▯

5. ⬠ is to ⬡

⬡ is to ?

a. ☐   b. ⯃

c. ⬠   d. ⬡

6. [⠿] is to [⠲]

[⠶] is to ?

a. [⠒⠂]   b. [⠿]

c. [⠔]   d. [⠢]

7. ▯ is to ▭

△ is to ?

a. ▷   b. ▭

c. ▷   d. ⬭

8. ◯ is to ()

☐ is to ?

a. ▫   b. ▯

c. ▭   d. ▫

9. Winner : Champion :: Sheen :

   a. Shimmer

   b. Dark

   c. Sweet

   d. Garbage

10. Frog : Amphibian :: Snake :

   a. Reptile

   b. Protozoan

   c. Mammals

   d. Bacteria

11. Petal : Flower :: Fur

   a. Coat

   b. Warm

   c. Woman

   d. Rabbit

12. Present : Birthday :: Reward :

   a. Accomplishment

   b. Medal

   c. acceptance

   d. cash

13. Shovel : Dig :: Scissors :

   a. Scoop

   b. Carry

   c. Snip

   d. Rip

14. Finger : Hand :: Leg :

    a. Body

    b. Foot

    c. Toe

    d. Hip

15. Sleep in : Late :: Skip breakfast :

    a. Hungry

    b. Early

    c. Lunch

    d. Dinner

16. Circle : Sphere :: Square :

    a. Triangle

    b. Oval

    c. Half Circle

    d. Cube

17. Orange : Fruit :: Carrot:

    a. Vegetable

    b. Bean

    c. Food

    d. Apple

18. Which of the following does not belong?

    a. ddeeffgg

    b. ffgghhii

    c. nnooppqq

    d. ttuuvvww

19. Which of the following does not belong?

    a. 11223344

    b. 33445566

    c. 33455666

    d. 44556677

20. Which of the following does not belong?

    a. mNo

    b. pQr

    c. Stu

    d. xYz

21. Which of the following does not belong?

    a. abcabc

    b. defdef

    c. ghihij

    d. mnomno

22. Which of the following does not belong?

    a. Dog

    b. Wolf

    c. Terrier

    d. Cougar

23. Which of the following does not belong?

    a. DDDdddEEE

    b. MMMoooPPP

    c. GGGhhhIII

    d. JJJkkkLLL

24. Which of the following does not belong?

a. cde

b. mno

c. stu

d. abc

25. Which of the following does not belong?

a. 446688

b. 224466

c. 336699

d. 66881010

26. Which of the following does not belong?

a. Assume

b. Certain

c. Sure

d. Positive

27. Which of the following does not belong?

a. MnOp

b. AbCD

c. QrSt

d. WxYz

28. Which of the following does not belong?

a. Look

b. See

c. Perceive

d. Surmise

29. Which of the following does not belong?

    a. Count

    b. Number

    c. Add up

    d. List

30. Which of the following does not belong?

    a. Secure

    b. Discard

    c. Throw out

    d. Abandon

Part II – Spelling

1. Choose the correct spelling.

    a. corespondence

    b. corespodence

    c. correspodence

    d. correspomdence

2. Choose the correct spelling.

    a. henmorrhage

    b. hemmorrhage

    c. hemorrhage

    d. hemorhage

3. Choose the correct spelling.

    a. enviromnment

    b. environment

    c. environiment

    d. enviromment

4. Choose the correct spelling.

a. govermment

b. goverment

c. govenment

d. government

5. Choose the correct spelling.

a. Conceeve

b. Concieve

c. Conceive

d. Conceve

6. Choose the correct spelling.

a. Describe

b. Decribe

c. Decsribe

d. Discribe

7. Choose the correct spelling.

a. Liqour

b. Liquor

c. Liquer

d. Liquour

8. Choose the correct spelling.

a. Succesful

b. Sucessful

c. Sucessfull

d. Successful

9. Choose the correct spelling.

    a. Huricane

    b. Hurricane

    c. Huricane

    d. Hurriccane

10. Choose the correct spelling.

    a. Precede

    b. Preccede

    c. Precceed

    d. Preceed

11. Choose the correct spelling.

    a. Embarasment

    b. Embarrasment

    c. Imbarrassment

    d. Embarrassment

12. Choose the correct spelling.

    a. Cutastrophy

    b. Catastrophe

    c. Catastrophy

    d. Catustrophy

13. Choose the correct spelling.

    a. Hygeine

    b. Hygiene

    c. Hygene

    d. None of the Above

14. Choose the correct spelling.

    a. Embellish

    b. Embelish

    c. Imbelish

    d. Embillesh

15. Choose the correct spelling.

    a. Previlige

    b. Prevelige

    c. Privilege

    d. Privelige

16. Choose the correct spelling.

    a. Stupendos

    b. Stupendous

    c. Stupendouos

    d. Stupendues

17. Choose the correct spelling.

    a. Obletireate

    b. Obletirate

    c. Oblitterate

    d. Obliterate

18. Choose the correct spelling.

    a. Miscellaeneus

    b. Miscellaneous

    c. Micellaneous

    d. Miscellaneouos

19. Choose the correct spelling.

a. Inoccuous

b. Ennocuous

c. Innoccuous

d. Innocuous

20. Choose the correct spelling.

a. Iminent

b. Emminent

c. Eminent

d. Iminennt

21. Choose the correct spelling.

a. Coalesque

b. Coalesce

c. Coalisque

d. Coalisque

22. Choose the correct spelling.

a. Bagage

b. Buggage

c. Baggage

d. Bugage

23. Choose the correct spelling.

a. Posible

b. Possible

c. Possibel

d. None of the Above

24. Choose the correct spelling.

    a. Pronounce

    b. Prononce

    c. Pronunce

    d. Pronounse

25. Choose the correct spelling.

    a. Accesible

    b. Acessible

    c. Acesible

    d. Accessible

26. Choose the correct spelling.

    a. Idiosyncracy

    b. Idiosyncrassy

    c. Idiosyncrasy

    d. Idiocyncrasy

27. Choose the correct spelling.

    a. Kechup

    b. Ketsup

    c. Kechup

    d. Ketchup

28. Choose the correct spelling.

    a. Maintainance

    b. Maintenace

    c. Maintanance

    d. Maintenance

29. Choose the correct spelling.

    a. Humoros

    b. Humouros

    c. Humorous

    d. Humorus

30. Choose the correct spelling.

    a. Knowlege

    b. knowledge

    c. Knowlegde

    d. Knowlledge

Section 1 – Reading Comprehension

Questions 1-4 refer to the following passage.

Passage 1 - The Respiratory System

The respiratory system's function is to allow oxygen exchange through all parts of the body. The anatomy or structure of the exchange system, and the uses of the exchanged gases, varies depending on the organism. In humans and other mammals, for example, the anatomical features of the respiratory system include airways, lungs, and the respiratory muscles. Molecules of oxygen and carbon dioxide are passively exchanged, by diffusion, between the gaseous external environment and the blood. This exchange process occurs in the alveolar region of the lungs.

Other animals, such as insects, have respiratory systems with very simple anatomical features, and in amphibians even the skin plays a vital role in gas exchange. Plants also have respiratory systems but the direction of gas exchange can be opposite to that of animals.

The respiratory system can also be divided into physiological, or functional, zones. These include the conducting zone (the region for gas transport from the outside atmosphere to just above the alveoli), the transitional zone, and the respiratory zone (the alveolar region where gas exchange occurs). [20]

1. What can we infer from the first paragraph in this passage?

    a. Human and mammal respiratory systems are the same

    b. The lungs are an important part of the respiratory system

    c. The respiratory system varies in different mammals

    d. Oxygen and carbon dioxide are passive exchanged by the respiratory system

2. What is the process by which molecules of oxygen and carbon dioxide are passively exchanged?

    a. Transfusion

    b. Affusion

    c. Diffusion

    d. Respiratory confusion

3. What organ plays an important role in gas exchange in amphibians?

    a. The skin

    b. The lungs

    c. The gills

    d. The mouth

4. What are the three physiological zones of the respiratory system?

    a. Conducting, transitional, respiratory zones

    b. Redacting, transitional, circulatory zones

    c. Conducting, circulatory, inhibiting zones

    d. Transitional, inhibiting, conducting zones

Questions 5-8 refer to the following passage.

ABC Electric Warranty

ABC Electric Company warrants that its products are free from defects in material and workmanship. Subject to the conditions and limitations set forth below, ABC Electric will, at its option, either repair or replace any part of its products that prove defective due to improper workmanship or materials.

This limited warranty does not cover any damage to the product from improper installation, accident, abuse, misuse, natural disaster, insufficient or excessive electrical supply, abnormal mechanical or environmental conditions, or any unauthorized disassembly, repair, or modification.

This limited warranty also does not apply to any product on which the original identification information has been altered, or removed, has not been handled or packaged correctly, or has been sold as second-hand.

This limited warranty covers only repair, replacement, refund or credit for defective ABC Electric products, as provided above.

5. I tried to repair my ABC Electric blender, but could not, so can I get it repaired under this warranty?

    a. Yes, the warranty still covers the blender

    b. No, the warranty does not cover the blender

    c. Uncertain. ABC Electric may or may not cover repairs under this warranty

6. My ABC Electric fan is not working. Will ABC Electric provide a new one or repair this one?

    a. ABC Electric will repair my fan

    b. ABC Electric will replace my fan

    c. ABC Electric could either replace or repair my fan can request either a replacement or a repair.

7. My stove was damaged in a flood. Does this warranty cover my stove?

    a. Yes, it is covered.

    b. No, it is not covered.

    c. It may or may not be covered.

    d. ABC Electric will decide if it is covered

8. Which of the following is an example of improper workmanship?

    a. Missing parts

    b. Defective parts

    c. Scratches on the front

    d. None of the above

Questions 9 – 11 refer to the following passage.

Passage 2 – Mythology

The main characters in myths are usually gods or supernatural heroes. As sacred stories, rulers and priests have traditionally endorsed their myths and as a result, myths have a close link with religion and politics. In the society where a myth originates, the natives believe the myth is a true account of the remote past. In fact, many societies have two categories of traditional narrative—(1) "true stories," or myths, and (2) "false stories," or fables.

Myths generally take place during a primordial age, when the world was still young, prior to achieving its current form. These stories explain how the world gained its current form and why the culture developed its customs, institutions, and taboos. Closely related to myth are legend and folktale. Myths, legends, and folktales are different types of traditional stories. Unlike myths, folktales can take place at any time and any place, and the natives do not usually consider them true or sacred. Legends, on the other hand, are similar to myths in that many people have traditionally considered them true. Legends take place in a more recent time, when the world was much as it is today. In addition, legends generally feature humans as their main characters, whereas myths have superhuman characters. [21]

9. We can infer from this passage that

a. Folktales took place in a time far past, before civilization covered the earth

b. Humankind uses myth to explain how the world was created

c. Myths revolve around gods or supernatural beings; the local community usually accepts these stories as not true

d. The only difference between a myth and a legend is the time setting of the story

10. The main purpose of this passage is

a. To distinguish between many types of traditional stories, and explain the back-ground of some traditional story categories

b. To determine whether myths and legends might be true accounts of history

c. To show the importance of folktales how these traditional stories made life more bearable in harder times

d. None of the Above

11. How are folktales different from myths?

    a.   Folktales and myth are the same

    b.   Folktales are not true and generally not sacred and take place anytime

    c.   Myths are not true and generally not sacred and take place anytime

    d.   Folktales explained the formation of the world and myths do not

Getting Started

12. Based on the partial Table of Contents above, what is this book about?

    a. How to answer multiple choice questions

    b. Different types of multiple choice questions

    c. How to write a test

    d. None of the above

Questions 13-16 refer to the following passage.

Passage 3 – Myths, Legend and Folklore

Cultural historians draw a distinction between myth, legend and folktale simply as a way to group traditional stories. However, in many cultures, drawing a sharp line between myths and legends is not that simple. Instead of dividing their traditional stories into myths, legends, and folktales, some cultures divide them into two categories. The first category roughly corresponds to folktales, and the second is one that combines myths and legends. Similarly, we cannot always separate myths from folktales. One society might consider a story true, making it a myth. Another society may believe the story is fiction, which makes it a folktale. In fact, when a myth loses its status as part of a religious system, it often takes on traits more typical of folktales, with its formerly divine characters now appearing as human heroes, giants, or fairies. Myth, legend, and folktale are only a few of the categories of traditional stories. Other categories include anecdotes and some kinds of jokes. Traditional stories, in turn, are only one category within the larger category of folklore, which also includes items such as gestures, costumes, and music. [21]

13. The main idea of this passage is

a. Myths, fables, and folktales are not the same thing, and each describes a specific type of story

b. Traditional stories can be categorized in different ways by different people

c. Cultures use myths for religious purposes, and when this is no longer true, the people forget and discard these myths

d. Myths can never become folk tales, because one is true, and the other is false

14. The terms myth and legend are

a. Categories that are synonymous with true and false

b. Categories that group traditional stories according to certain characteristics

c. Interchangeable, because both terms mean a story that is passed down from generation to generation

d. Meant to distinguish between a story that involves a hero and a cultural message and a story meant only to entertain

15. Traditional story categories not only include myths and legends, but

a. Can also include gestures, since some cultures passed these down before the written and spoken word

b. In addition, folklore refers to stories involving fables and fairy tales

c. These story categories can also include folk music and traditional dress

d. Traditional stories themselves are a part of the larger category of folklore, which may also include costumes, gestures, and music

16. This passage shows that

a. There is a distinct difference between a myth and a legend, although both are folktales

b. Myths are folktales, but folktales are not myths

c. Myths, legends, and folktales play an important part in tradition and the past, and are a rich and colorful part of history

d. Most cultures consider myths to be true

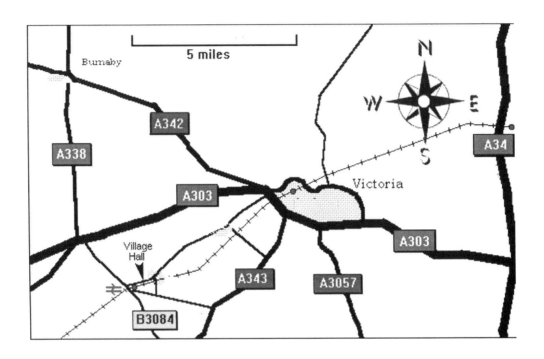

17. Approximately how far is Victoria to Burnaby?

a. About 10 miles

b. About 5 miles

c. About 15 miles

d. About 20 miles

18. How is the Village Hall from Victoria?

a. About 10 miles

b. About 5 miles

c. About 15 miles

d. About 20 miles

Questions 19 - 23 refer to the following passage.

Passage 4 – Trees I

Trees are an important part of the natural landscape because they prevent erosion and protect ecosystems in and under their branches. Trees also play an important role in producing oxygen and reducing carbon dioxide in the atmosphere, as well as moderating ground temperatures. Trees are important elements in landscaping and agriculture, both for their visual appeal and for their crops, such as apples, and other fruit. Wood from trees is a building material, and a primary energy source in many developing countries. Trees also play a role in many of the world's mythologies. [22]

19. What are two reasons trees are important in the natural landscape?

    a. They prevent erosion and produce oxygen

    b. They produce fruit and are important elements in landscaping

    c. Trees are not important in the natural landscape

    d. Trees produce carbon dioxide and prevent erosion

20. What kind of ecosystems do trees protect?

    a. Trees do not protect ecosystems

    b. Weather sheltered ecosystems

    c. Ecosystems around the base and under the branches

    d. All of the above

21. Which of the following is true?

    a. Trees provide a primary food source in the developing world

    b. Trees provide a primary building material in the developing world

    c. Trees provide a primary energy source in the developing world

    d. Trees provide a primary oxygen source in the developing world

22. Why are trees important for agriculture?

    a. Because of their crops

    b. Because they shelter ecosystems

    c. Because they are a source of energy

    d. Because of their visual appeal

23. What do trees do to the atmosphere?

    a. Trees produce carbon dioxide and reduce oxygen

    b. Trees product oxygen and carbon dioxide

    c. Trees reduce oxygen and carbon dioxide

    d. Trees produce oxygen and reduce carbon dioxide

Questions 24 - 27 refer to the following passage.

Passage 5 – The Life of Helen Keller

Many people have heard of Helen Keller. She is famous because she was unable to see or hear, but learned to speak and read and went onto attend college and earn a degree. Her life is a very interesting story, one that she developed into an autobiography, which was then adapted into both a stage play and a movie. How did Helen Keller overcome her disabilities to become a famous woman? Read onto find out.

Helen Keller was not born blind and deaf. When she was a small baby, she had a very high fever for several days. As a result of her sudden illness, baby Helen lost her eyesight and her hearing. Because she was so young when she went deaf and blind, Helen Keller never had any recollection of being able to see or hear. Since she could not hear, she could not learn to talk. Since she could not see, it was difficult for her to move around. For the first six years of her life, her world was very still and dark.

Imagine what Helen's childhood must have been like. She could not hear her mother's voice. She could not see the beauty of her parent's farm. She could not recognize who was giving her a hug, or a bath or even where her bedroom was each night. More sad, she could not communicate with her parents in any way. She could not express her feelings or tell them the things she wanted. It must have been a very sad childhood.

When Helen was six years old, her parents hired her a teacher named Anne Sullivan. Anne was a young woman who was almost blind. However, she could hear and she could read Braille, so she was a perfect teacher for young Helen. At first, Anne had a very hard time teaching Helen anything. She described her first impression of Helen as a "wild thing, not a child." Helen did not like Anne at first either. She bit and hit Anne when Anne tried to teach her. However, the two of them eventually came to have a great deal of love and respect.

Anne taught Helen to hear by putting her hands on people's throats. She could feel the sounds that people made. In time, Helen learned to feel what people said. Next, Anne taught Helen to read Braille, which is a way that books are written for the blind. Finally, Anne taught Helen to talk. Although Helen did learn to talk, it was hard for anyone but Anne to understand her.

As Helen grew older, more and more people were amazed by her story. She went to college and wrote books about her life. She gave talks to the public, with Anne at her side, translating her words. Today, both Anne Sullivan and Helen Keller are famous women who are respected for their lives' work.

24. Helen Keller could not see and hear and so, what was her biggest problem in childhood?

  a. Inability to communicate

  b. Inability to walk

  c. Inability to play

  d. Inability to eat

25. Helen learned to hear by feeling the vibrations people made when they spoke. What were these vibrations were felt through?

  a. Mouth

  b. Throat

  c. Ears

  d. Lips

26. From the passage, we can infer that Anne Sullivan was a patient teacher. We can infer this because

  a. Helen hit and bit her and Anne still remained her teacher.

  b. Anne taught Helen to read only.

  c. Anne was hard of hearing too.

  d. Anne wanted to be a teacher.

27. Helen Keller learned to speak but Anne translated her words when she spoke in public. The reason Helen needed a translator was because

  a. Helen spoke another language.

  b. Helen's words were hard for people to understand.

  c. Helen spoke very quietly.

  d. Helen did not speak but only used sign language.

Questions 28 - 30 refer to the following passage.

Lowest Price Guarantee

Get it for less. Guaranteed!

ABC Electric will beat any advertised price by 10% of the difference.

  1) If you find a lower advertised price, we will beat it by 10% of the difference.

2) If you find a lower advertised price within 30 days* of your purchase we will beat it by 10% of the difference.

3) If our own price is reduced within 30 days* of your purchase, bring in your receipt and we will refund the difference.

*14 days for computers, monitors, printers, laptops, tablets, cellular & wireless devices, home security products, projectors, camcorders, digital cameras, radar detectors, portable DVD players, DJ and pro-audio equipment, and air conditioners.

28. I bought a radar detector 15 days ago and saw an ad for the same model only cheaper. Can I get 10% of the difference refunded?

a. Yes. Since it is less than 30 days, you can get 10% of the difference refunded.

b. No. Since it is more than 14 days, you cannot get 10% of the difference re-funded.

c. It depends on the cashier.

d. Yes. You can get the difference refunded.

29. I bought a flat-screen TV for $500 10 days ago and found an advertisement for the same TV, at another store, on sale for $400. How much will ABC refund under this guarantee?

a. $100

b. $110

c. $10

d. $400

30. What is the purpose of this passage?

a. To inform

b. To educate

c. To persuade

d. To entertain

Questions 31 - 33 refer to the following passage.

Passage 6 - What Is Mardi Gras?

Mardi Gras is fast becoming one of the South's most famous and most celebrated holidays. The word Mardi Gras comes from the French and the literal translation is "Fat Tuesday." The holiday has also been called Shrove Tuesday, due to its associations with Lent. The purpose of Mardi Gras is to celebrate and enjoy before the Lenten season of fasting and repentance begins.

What originated by the French Explorers in New Orleans, Louisiana in the 17th century is now celebrated all over the world. Panama, Italy, Belgium and Brazil all host large scale Mardi Gras celebrations, and many smaller cities and towns celebrate this fun loving Tuesday as well. Usually held in February or early March, Mardi Gras is a day of extravagance, a day for people to eat, drink and be merry, to wear costumes, masks and to dance to jazz music.
The French explorers on the Mississippi River would be in shock today if they saw the opulence of the parades and floats that grace the New Orleans streets during Mardi Gras these days. Parades in New Orleans are divided by organizations. These are more commonly known as Krewes.

Being a member of a Krewe is quite a task because Krewes are responsible for overseeing the parades. Each Krewe's parade is ruled by a Mardi Gras "King and Queen." The role of the King and Queen is to "bestow" gifts on their adoring fans as the floats ride along the street. They throw doubloons, which is fake money and usually colored green, purple and gold, which are the colors of Mardi Gras. Beads in those color shades are also thrown and cups are thrown as well. Beads are by far the most popular souvenir of any Mardi Gras parade, with each spectator attempting to gather as many as possible.

31. The purpose of Mardi Gras is to

    a. Repent for a month.

    b. Celebrate in extravagant ways.

    c. Be a member of a Krewe.

    d. Explore the Mississippi.

32. From reading the passage we can infer that "Kings and Queens"

    a. Have to be members of a Krewe.

    b. Have to be French.

    c. Have to know how to speak French.

    d. Have to give away their own money.

33. Which group of people first began to hold Mardi Gras celebrations?

    a. Settlers from Italy

    b. Members of Krewes

    c. French explorers

    d. Belgium explorers

Questions 33-35 refer to the following passage.

Passage 7 - The Circulatory System

The circulatory system is an organ system that passes nutrients (such as amino acids and electrolytes), gases, hormones, and blood cells to and from cells in the body to help fight diseases and help stabilize body temperature and pH levels.

The circulatory system may be seen strictly as a blood distribution network, but some consider the circulatory system as composed of the cardiovascular system, which distributes blood, and the lymphatic system, which distributes lymph. While humans, as well as other vertebrates, have a closed cardiovascular system (meaning that the blood never leaves the network of arteries, veins and capillaries), some invertebrate groups have an open cardiovascular system. The most primitive animal phyla lack circulatory systems. The lymphatic system, on the other hand, is an open system.

Two types of fluids move through the circulatory system: blood and lymph. The blood, heart, and blood vessels form the cardiovascular system. The lymph, lymph nodes, and lymph vessels form the lymphatic system. The cardiovascular system and the lymphatic system collectively make up the circulatory system.

The main components of the human cardiovascular system are the heart and the blood vessels. It includes: the pulmonary circulation, a "loop" through the lungs where blood is oxygenated; and the systemic circulation, a "loop" through the rest of the body to provide oxygenated blood. An average adult contains five to six quarts (roughly 4.7 to 5.7 liters) of blood, which consists of plasma, red blood cells, white blood cells, and platelets. Also, the digestive system works with the circula-

tory system to provide the nutrients the system needs to keep the heart pumping.
[22]

33. What can we infer from the first paragraph?

a. An important purpose of the circulatory system is that of fighting diseases.

b. The most important function of the circulatory system is to give the person energy.

c. The least important function of the circulatory system is that of growing skin cells.

d. The entire purpose of the circulatory system is not known.

34. Do humans have an open or closed circulatory system?

a. Open

b. Closed

c. Usually open, though sometimes closed

d. Usually closed, though sometimes open

35. In addition to blood, what two components form the cardiovascular system?

a. The heart and the lungs

b. The lungs and the veins

c. The heart and the blood vessels

d. The blood vessels and the nerves

Section IV – Basic Science

1. Which of the following is not true:

a. Genotypes are inherited information

b. Phenotypes are inherited information

c. Phenotypes are observed behavior

d. Phenotypes include an organisms development

2. Electrons play a critical role in:

    a. Electricity

    b. Magnetism

    c. Thermal conductivity

    d. All of the above

3. An idea concerning a phenomena and possible explanations for that phenomena is a/an

    a. Theory

    b. Experiment

    c. Inference

    d. Hypothesis

4. Define chromosomes.

    a. Structures in a cell nucleus that carry genetic material.

    b. Consist of thousands of DNA strands.

    c. Total 46 in a normal human cell.

    d. all of the above

5. What is one of the best known disorders that attack the immune system?

    a. Rabies

    b. HIV

    c. Lung cancer

    d. Muscular dystrophy

6. Which disease of the circulatory system is one of the most frequent causes of death in North America?

    a. The cold

    b. Pneumonia

    c. Arthritis

    d. Heart disease

7. Which of the following describes a plasma membrane?

a. Lipids with embedded proteins

b. An outer lipid layer and an inner lipid layer

c. Proteins embedded in lipid bilayer

d. Altering protein and lipid layers

8. What is the difference between Strong Nuclear Force and Weak Nuclear Force?

a. The Strong Nuclear Force is an attractive force that binds protons and neutrons and maintains the structure of the nucleus, and the Weak Nuclear Force is responsible for the radioactive beta decay and other subatomic reactions.

b. The Strong Nuclear Force is responsible for the radioactive beta decay and other subatomic reactions, and the Weak Nuclear Force is an attractive force that binds protons and neutrons and maintains the structure of the nucleus.

c. The Weak Nuclear Force is feeble and the Strong Nuclear Force is robust.

d. The Strong Nuclear Force is a negative force that releases protons and neutrons and threatens the structure of the nucleus, and the Weak Nuclear Force is an attractive force that binds protons and neutrons and maintains the structure of the nucleus.

9. What type of research deals with the quality, type or components of a group, substance, or mixture.

a. Quantitative

b. Dependent

c. Scientific

d. Qualitative

10. Adaptation is:

a. A trait that has evolved by natural selection

b. A trait that has been bred by artificial selection

c. A trait that has no function in an organism

d. None of the above

11. Describe a pH indicator.

a. A pH indicator measures hydrogen ions in a solution and show pH on a color scale.

b. A pH indicator measures oxygen ions in a solution and show pH on a color scale.

c. A pH indicator many different types of ions in a solution and shows pH on a color scale

d. None of the above

12. What is the earth's primary source of energy?

a. Water

b. The sun

c. Electromagnetic radiation

d. Weak nuclear force

13. What type of research is to determine the relationship between one thing (an independent variable) and another (a dependent or outcome variable) in a population.

a. Qualitative

b. Quantitative

c. Independent

d. Scientific

14. What can accept a hydrogen ion and can react with fats to form soaps?

a. Acid

b. Salt

c. Base

d. Foundation

15. Which gene, whose presence as a single copy, controls the expression of a trait?

a. Principal gene

b. Latent gene

c. Recessive gene

d. Dominant gene

16. Within taxonomy, plants and animals are considered two basic _____.

    a. Families

    b. Kingdoms

    c. Domains

    d. Genus

17. Organisms grouped into the _____ Kingdom include all unicellular organisms lacking a definite cellular arrangement such as _____ and _____.

    a. Fungi, bacteria, algae

    b. Protista, bacteria, amphibian

    c. Protista, bacteria, algae

    d. Plantae, bacteria, algae

18. What is a common digestive affliction that most people suffer at one time or other?

    a. Stomach cancer

    b. Ulceritis

    c. Indigestion

    d. The flu

19. What are the biochemical and biophysical activities that all living systems must be able to carry out to maintain life?

    a. Life sequences

    b. Life expectancies

    c. Life cycles

    d. Life functions

20. What disease of the circulatory system is often mistaken for a heart attack?

    a. Cardiac arrest

    b. High blood pressure

    c. Angina

    d. Acid reflux

21. Define a biological class.

   a. A collection of similar or like living entities.

   b. Two or more animals in a group, all having the same parent.

   c. All animals sharing the same living environment.

   d. All plant life that share the same physical properties.

22. What type of foods that stay in the stomach longest?

   a. Fats

   b. Proteins

   c. Carbohydrates

   d. Vitamins

23. How many elements are represented on the periodic table?

   a. 122 elements

   b. 99 elements

   c. 102 elements

   d. 118 elements

24. What is the diagram that is used to predict an outcome of a particular cross or breeding experiment?

   a. Genetic puzzle

   b. Genome project

   c. Hybrid theorem

   d. Punnett square

25. Which, if any, of the following statements about prokaryotic cells is false?

   a. Prokaryotic cells include such organisms as E. coli and Streptococcus.

   b. Prokaryotic cells lack internal membranes and organelles.

   c. Prokaryotic cells break down food using cellular respiration and fermentation.

   d. All of these statements are true.

26. What is the process of converting observed phenomena into data is called?

  a. Calculation

  b. Measurement

  c. Valuation

  d. Estimation

27. The mass number of an atom is:

  a. The total number of particles that make it up

  b. The total weight of an atom

  c. The total mass of an atom

  d. None of the above

28. What is sublimation?

  a. A phase transition from liquid to gas

  b. A phase transition from solid to gas

  c. A phase transition from gas to liquid

  d. A phase transition from gas to solid

29. How is exhalation accomplished?

  a. By the abdominal muscles

  b. By the chest muscles

  c. By the esophagus

  d. By the nasal passageway

30. What three processes are involved in cell division of Eukaryotic cells?

  a. Meiosis, cytokinesis, and interphase

  b. Meiosis, mitosis, and interphase

  c. Mitosis, kinematisis, and interphase

  d. Mitosis, cytokinesis, and interphase

31. Describe genotypes.

a. The genetic makeup, as distinguished from the physical appearance, of an organism or a group of organisms.

b. The combination of alleles located on homologous chromosomes that determines a specific characteristic or trait.

c. Is the inheritable information carried by all living organisms.

d. All of the above.

32. What does the respiratory system primarily oxygenate?

a. The brain

b. The limbs

c. The heart

d. The blood

33. What chain of nucleotides plays an important role in the creation of new proteins?

a. Deoxyribonucleic acid (DNA) is a chain of nucleotides that plays an important role in the creation of new proteins.

b. Ribonucleic acid (RNA) is a chain of nucleotides that plays an important role in the creation of new proteins.

c. There are no chains of nucleotides that play a role in the creation of proteins.

d. None of the above.

34. A practical test designed with the intention that its results will be relevant to a particular theory or set of theories is a/an

a. Experiment

b. Practicum

c. Theory

d. Design

35. Strong chemical bonds include

a. Dipole - dipole interactions

b. Hydrogen bonding

c. Covalent or ionic bonds

d. None of the above

36. What is the process that the immune system adapts over time to be more efficient in recognizing pathogens?

a. Acquired immunity

b. AIDS

c. Pathogens

d. Acquired deficiency

37. What is a group of tissues that perform a specific function or group of functions?

a. System

b. Tissue

c. Group

d. Organ

38. What is the measure of an experiment's ability to yield the same or compatible results in different clinical experiments or statistical trials?

a. Variability

b. Validity

c. Control measure

d. Reliability

39. Describe each chemical element in the periodic table.

a. Each chemical element has a unique atomic number representing the number of electrons in its nucleus.

b. Each chemical element has a varying atomic number depending on the number of protons in its nucleus.

c. Each chemical element has a unique atomic number representing the number of protons in its nucleus.

d. None of the above.

40. The immune system is

a. The system that expels waste from the body.

b. The system that expels carbon dioxide from the body.

c. The system that protects the body from disease and infection.

d. The system that circulates blood through the body.

41. The binding membrane of an animal cell is called

a. The biological membrane

b. The cell coat

c. The unit membrane

d. The plasma membrane

42. Define organelles

a. A protein in a cell

b. An enzyme in a cell

c. A specialized subunit of a cell with a specific function

d. A cell membrane

43. A solution with a pH value of less than 7 is

a. Acid solution

b. Base solution

c. Neutral pH solution

d. None of the above

44. Is a catalyst changed by a reaction?

a. Yes

b. No

c. It may be changed depending on the other chemicals

45. The _____ is the prediction that an observed difference is due to chance alone and not due to a systematic cause; this hypothesis is tested by statistical analysis, and either accepted or rejected.

    a. Null hypothesis

    b. Hypothesis

    c. Control

    d. Variable

46. In science, industry, and statistics, the _____ of a measurement system is the degree of closeness of measurements of a quantity to its actual (true) value.

    a. Mistake

    b. Uncertainty

    c. Accuracy

    d. Error

47. What is a more common name for the circulatory system disease known as hypertension?

    a. Anemia

    b. High blood pressure

    c. Angina

    d. Cardiac arrest

48. The ___ of a distribution is the difference between the maximum value and the minimum value.

    a. Distribution

    b. Range

    c. Mode

    d. Median

49. What is a statistical technique which determines if two variables are related.

a. Statistical correlation

b. Statistical measurement

c. Control group

d. Statistical analysis

50. What is the mathematical average of a set of numbers.

a. Mean

b. Median

c. Distribution

d. Standard deviation

51. What is the simplest unit of any compound?

a. Atom

b. Proton

c. Molecule

d. Compound

52. What results when acid reacts with a base?

a. A weak acid

b. A weak base

c. A salt and water

d. Hydrogen

53. The horizontal rows of the periodic table are known as

a. Groups

b. Periods

c. Series

d. Columns

54. When do oxidation and reduction reactions occur?

    a. One after the other

    b. In separate reactions

    c. On the product side of the reaction

    d. Simultaneously

55. What are most of the elements on the periodic table classified as?

    a. Nonmetals

    b. Metals

    c. Metalloids

    d. Gases

56. What is usually the result when acid reacts with most of the metals?

    a. Carbon dioxide

    b. Oxygen gas

    c. Nitrogen gas

    d. Hydrogen gas

57. What are the vertical columns of the periodic table?

    a. Series

    b. Groups

    c. Periods

    d. Columns

58. In a redox reaction, how many electrons are lost?

    a. Less than the number of electrons gained

    b. More than the number of electrons gained

    c. Equal to the number of electrons gained

    d. None of the above

59. A substance containing atoms of more than one element in a definite ratio is called a(n)

   a. Compound

   b. Element

   c. Mixture

   d. Molecule

60. All acids turn blue litmus paper

   a. Blue

   b. Red

   c. Green

   d. White

Answer Key

Part 1 Academic Aptitude

Vocabulary

1. D
2. A
3. D
4. C
5. D
6. A
7. A
8. B
9. D
10. A
11. B
12. C
13. B
14. C
15. A
16. C
17. D
18. C
19. D
20. B
21. A
22. D
23. D
24. C
25. D
26. C
27. A
28. B
29. C
30. C

Mathematics

1. D
We understand that each of the n employees earn s amount of salary weekly. This means that one employee earns s salary weekly. So; Richard has ns amount of money to employ n employees for a week.

We are asked to find the number of days n employees can be employed with x amount of money. We can do simple direct proportion:

If Richard can employ n employees for 7 days with ns amount of money,

Richard can employ n employees for y days with x amount of money ... y is the number of days we need to find.

We can do cross multiplication:

y = (x•7)/(ns)

y = 7x/ns

2. A
Five greater than 3 times a number.
5 + 3 times a number.
3X + 5

3. C
MMXIII is 2013. 1,000 + 1,000 + 10 + 1 + 1 + 1.

4. D
x2 + 4x = 5, x2 + 4x - 5 = 0, x2 + 5x - x - 5 = 0, factorize x(x + 5) -1(x + 5) = o, (x + 5)(x - 1) = 0. x + 5 = 0 or x - 1 = 0, x = 0 - 5 or x = 0 + 1, x = -5 or x = 1, either b or c.

5. A
The number is 51.738. The last digit, in the 1,000th place, 2, is less than 5, so it is discarded. Answer = 765.368.

6. D
This is a simple direct proportion problem:
If Lynn can type 1 page in p minutes,

   she can type x pages in 5 minutes

We do cross multiplication: x•p = 5•1

Then,

x = 5/p

7. A
This is an inverse ration problem.

1/x = 1/a + 1/b where a is the time Sally can paint a house, b is the time John can paint a house, x is the time Sally and John can together paint a house.

So,

1/x = 1/4 + 1/6 ... We use the least common multiple in the denominator that is 24:

1/x = 6/24 + 4/24

1/x = 10/24

x = 24/10

x = 2.4 hours.

In other words; 2 hours + 0.4 hours = 2 hours + 0.4•60 minutes

= 2 hours 24 minutes

8. D
The cost of the dishwasher = $450

15% discount amount = 450•15/100 = $67.5

The discounted price = 450 – 67.5 = $382.5

20% additional discount amount on lowest price = 382.5•20/100 = $76.5

So, the final discounted price = 382.5 - 76.5 = $306.00

9. D
Original price = x,
80/100 = 12590/X,
80X = 1259000,
X = 15,737.50.

10. A
25% = 25/100 = 1/4

11. C
125/100 = 1.25

12. C
24/56 = 3/7 (divide numerator and denominator by 8)

13. C
Converting a fraction into a decimal – divide the numerator by the denominator – so 71/1000 = .071. Dividing by 1000 moves the decimal point 3 places to the left.

14. C
9 is in the ten thousandths place in 1.7389, which is 4 places to the right of the decimal point.

15. A
(6-4) (3/5 – 4/5) = 2 (3-4/5) = since 3 is less than 4, we would have to subtract 1 from the whole number besides the fraction, therefore 1 13-4/5 = 1 9/5 = 2 4/5

16. A
Step 1: Set up the formula to calculate the dose to be given in mg as per weight of the child:-
Dose ordered X Weight in Kg = Dose to be given
Step 2: 100 mg X 23 kg = 2300 mg
(Convert 50 lb to Kg, 1 lb = 0.4536 kg, hence 50 lb = 50 X 0.4536 = 22.68 kg approx. 23 kg)
2300 mg/230 mg X 1 tablet/1 = 2300/230 = 10 tablets

17. D
To find the total turnout in all three polling stations, we need to proportion the number of voters to the number of all registered voters.

Number of total voters = 945 + 860 + 1210 = 3015

Number of total registered voters = 1270 + 1050 + 1440 = 3760

Percentage turnout over all three polling stations = 3015•100/3760 = 80.19%

Checking the answers, we round 80.19 to the nearest whole number: 80%

18. D
600 mg/ 200 mg X 1 tablet/1 = 600/200 = 3 tablets

19. C
At 100% efficiency 1 machine produces 1450/10 = 145 m of cloth.

At 95% efficiency, 4 machines produce 4•145•95/100 = 551 m of cloth.

At 90% efficiency, 6 machines produce 6•145•90/100 = 783 m of cloth.

Total cloth produced by all 10 machines = 551 + 783 = 1334 m

Since the information provided and the question are based on 8 hours, we did not need to use time to reach the answer.

20. C
1 foot = 12 inches, 60 feet = 60 x 12 = 720 inches.

21. A
The ratio between black and blue pens is 7 to 28 or 7:28. Bring to the lowest terms by dividing both sides by 7 gives 1:4.

22. A
1 millimeter = 10 centimeter, 100 millimeter = 100/10 = 10 centimeters.

23. C
1 gallon = 4 quarts, 3 gallons = 3 x 4 = 12 quarts.

24. D
1 inch on map = 2,000 inches on ground. So, 5.2 inches on map = 5.2•2,000 = 10,400 inches on ground.

25. B
There are 1000 ml in a liter. 0.05/1000 = 0.00005 liters.

26. D
X% of 120 = 30,
X/100 = 10/120
so X = 30/120 x 100/1
3000/120 = 300/12
X = 25

27. B
There are 52 cards in total. Smith has 16 cards in which he can win. Therefore, his probability of winning in a single game will be 16/52. Simon has 20 winning cards so his probability of winning in single draw is 20/52.

28. A
There are 100 centimeters in a meter, so 100 X .45 meters = 45 centimeters.

29. A
Based on this graph, a person that is 85 will make 26.2 visits to the hospital every year.

30. C
A person aged 95 or older would make more than 31.3 visits.

Nonverbal

1. A

The relation is the same figure rotated.

2. D

The relation is the same figure rotated.

3. B

The relation is a 3-dimensional figure to a 2-dimensional figure.

4. B

The relation is a 2-dimensional figure to a 3-dimensional figure.

5. B

The relation is a n-sided figure to an n+1 sided figure.

6. C

The first figure has 9 cots in a square and the second figure has 6 dots, which is 1/3 removed.

7. C

The relation is a 3-dimentional figure to a rotated 2-dimentional figure.

8. C

The relation is the same figure with the bottom half removed.

9. A

This is a synonym relationship. Shimmer has the same meaning as sheen.

10. A

This is a classification relationship. Reptile is the classification taxa for snake.

11. D

This is a part-to-whole relationship. A petal is to a flower as fur is to a rabbit.

12. A

A present celebrates a birthday and a reward celebrates an accomplishment.

13. C

This is a functional relationship. A shovel is used to dig and scissors are used to snip.

14. A

This is a parts-to-whole relationship. The finger is part of the hand in the same way a leg is part of a body.

15. A
This is a cause and effect relationship. If you sleep in you will be late. If you skip breakfast, you will be hungry.

16. D
A sphere is the solid form of a circle just as a cube is the solid form of a square.

17. A
This is a classification relationship. An orange is a fruit and a carrot is a vegetable.

18. B
This is a vowel and consonant relationship. All the choices have vowels in positions 3 and 4.

19. C
This is a repetition pattern. All the choices have consecutive numbers repeated twice.

20. C
This is a capital to small letter relationship. All choices have the middle letter capitalized.

21. C
This is a repetition pattern. All the choices repeat a three number sequence.

22. D
This is a relationship of words question. All the choices are dog or canine family except cougar.

23. B
This is a repetition pattern. All the choices repeat consecutive 3-number patterns.

24. D
This is a vowel and consonant relationship. All the choices have a vowel at the end.

25. C
This is a repetition pattern. All the choices repeat a 2-letter sequence obtained by adding two to the previous number.

26. A

This is a word meaning relationship. Assume is not a synonym for any of the choices.

27. B

This is a capital small letter relationship. All choices have alternate letters capitalized.

28. D

This is a relationship of words question. All the choices are synonyms of look and see, except surmise.

29. D

This is a word meaning relationship. List is not a synonym for any of the choices.

30. A

All of choices are synonyms of discard except secure.

Part II – Spelling

1. A
2. C
3. B
4. D
5. C
6. A
7. B
8. D
9. B
10. A
11. D
12. B
13. B
14. A
15. C
16. B
17. D
18. B
19. D
20. C
21. B
22. C

23. B
24. A
25. D
26. C
27. D
28. D
29. C
30. B

Part III Reading Comprehension

1. B
We can infer an important part of the respiratory system are the lungs. From the passage, "Molecules of oxygen and carbon dioxide are passively exchanged, by diffusion, between the gaseous external environment and the blood. This exchange process occurs in the alveolar region of the lungs."

Therefore, one of the primary functions for the respiratory system is the exchange of oxygen and carbon dioxide, and this process occurs in the lungs. We can therefore infer that the lungs are an important part of the respiratory system.

2. C
The process by which molecules of oxygen and carbon dioxide are passively exchanged is diffusion.

This is a definition type question. Scan the passage for references to "oxygen," "carbon dioxide," or "exchanged."

3. A
The organ that plays an important role in gas exchange in amphibians is the skin.

Scan the passage for references to "amphibians," and find the answer.

4. A
The three physiological zones of the respiratory system are Conducting, transitional, respiratory zones.

5. B
This warranty does not cover a product that you have tried to fix yourself. From paragraph two, "This limited warranty does not cover ... any unauthorized disassembly, repair, or modification. "

6. C
ABC Electric could either replace or repair the fan, provided the other conditions are met. ABC Electric has the option to repair or replace.

7. B

The warranty does not cover a stove damaged in a flood. From the passage, "This limited warranty does not cover any damage to the product from improper installation, accident, abuse, misuse, natural disaster, insufficient or excessive electrical supply, abnormal mechanical or environmental conditions."

A flood is an "abnormal environmental condition," and a natural disaster, so it is not covered.

8. A

A missing part is an example of defective workmanship. This is an error made in the manufacturing process. A defective part is not considered workmanship.

9. B

The first paragraph tells us that myths are a true account of the remote past.

The second paragraph tells us that, "myths generally take place during a primordial age, when the world was still young, before achieving its current form."

Putting these two together, we can infer that humankind used myth to explain how the world was created.

10. A

This passage is about different types of stories. First, the passage explains myths, and then compares other types of stories to myths.

11. B

From the passage, "Unlike myths, folktales can take place at any time and any place, and the natives do not usually consider them true or sacred."

12. A

Based on the partial table of contents, this book is most likely about how to answer multiple choice.

13. B

This passage describes the different categories for traditional stories. The other choices are facts from the passage, not the main idea of the passage. The main idea of a passage will always be the most general statement. For example, choice A, Myths, fables, and folktales are not the same thing, and each describes a specific type of story. This is a true statement from the passage, but not the main idea of the passage, since the passage also talks about how some cultures may classify a story as a myth and others as a folktale.

The statement, from choice B, Traditional stories can be categorized in different ways by different people, is a more general statement that describes the passage.

14. B

Choice B is the best choice, categories that group traditional stories according to certain characteristics.

Choices A and C are false and can be eliminated right away. Choice D is designed to confuse. Choice D may be true, but it is not mentioned in the passage.

15. D
The best answer is D, traditional stories themselves are a part of the larger category of folklore, which may also include costumes, gestures, and music.

All of the other choices are false. Traditional stories are part of the larger category of Folklore, which includes other things, not the other way around.

16. A
There is a distinct difference between a myth and a legend, although both are folktales.

17. A
Victoria is about 5 miles from Burnaby.

18. B
The Village Hall is about 5 miles from Victoria.

19. A
Choice A is a re-wording of text from the passage.

20. C
This is taken directly from the passage.

21. C
Although trees are used as a building material, this is not their primary use. Trees are a primary energy source.

22. A
This is taken directly from the passage.

23. D
This question is designed to confuse by presenting different choices for the two chemicals, oxygen and carbon dioxide. One is produced, and one is reduced. Read the passage carefully to see which is reduced and which is produced.

24. B
The correct answer because that fact is stated directly in the passage. The passage explains that Anne taught Helen to hear by allowing her to feel the vibrations in her throat.

25. A
We can infer that Anne is a patient teacher because she did not leave or lose her

temper when Helen bit or hit her; she just kept trying to teach Helen. Choice B is incorrect because Anne taught Helen to read and talk. Choice C is incorrect because Anne could hear. She was partially blind, not deaf. Choice D is incorrect because it does not have to do with patience.

26. B

The passage states that it was hard for anyone but Anne to understand Helen when she spoke. Choice A is incorrect because the passage does not mention Helen spoke a foreign language. Choice C is incorrect because there is no mention of how quiet or loud Helen's voice was. Choice D is incorrect because we know from reading the passage that Helen did learn to speak.

27. D

This question tests the reader's summarization skills. The other choices A, B, and C focus on portions of the second paragraph that are too narrow and do not relate to the specific portion of text in question. The complexity of the sentence may mislead students into selecting one of these answers, but rearranging or restating the sentence will lead the reader to the correct answer. In addition, choice A makes an assumption that may or may not be true about the intentions of the company, choice B focuses on one product rather than the idea of the products, and choice C makes an assumption about women that may or may not be true and is not supported by the text.

28. B

The time limit for radar detectors is 14 days. Since you made the purchase 15 days ago, you do not qualify for the guarantee.

29. B

Since you made the purchase 10 days ago, you are covered by the guarantee. Since it is an advertised price at a different store, ABC Electric will "beat" the price by 10% of the difference, which is,

500 – 400 = 100 – difference in price

100 X 10% = $10 – 10% of the difference

The advertised lower price is $400. ABC will beat this price by 10% so they will refund $100 + 10 = $110.

30. C

The purpose of this passage is to persuade.

31. B

The correct answer can be found in the fourth sentence of the first paragraph.

Option A is incorrect because repenting begins the day AFTER Mardi Gras. Option C is incorrect because you can celebrate Mardi Gras without being a member of a Krewe.

Option D is incorrect because exploration does not play any role in a modern Mardi Gras celebration.

32. A
The second sentence is the last paragraph states that Krewes are led by the Kings and Queens. Therefore, you must have to be part of a Krewe to be its King or its Queen.

Option B is incorrect because it never states in the passage that only people from France can be Kings and Queen of Mardi Gras. Option C is incorrect because the passage says nothing about having to speak French. Option D is incorrect because the passage does state that the Kings and Queens throw doubloons, which is fake money.

33. C
The first sentences of BOTH the 2nd and 3rd paragraphs mention that French explorers started this tradition in New Orleans.

34. B
Humans have an closed circulatory system.

35. C
Besides blood, the heart and the blood vessels form the cardiovascular system.

Section IV – Basic Science

1. B
The only statement that is NOT true is, Phenotypes are inherited information.

2. D
All of the above are true. Electrons play an essential role in electricity, magnetism, and thermal conductivity.

3. D
An idea concerning a phenomena and possible explanations for that phenomena is an hypothesis.

4. D
All of the above

a. Structures in a cell nucleus that carry genetic material.
b. Consist of thousands of DNA strands.
c. Total 46 in a normal human cell.

5. B
One of the best known disorders that attack the immune system is HIV (the virus that causes AIDS).

6. D
The circulatory system disease that is one of the most frequent causes of death in North America is heart disease.

7. C
The plasma membrane or cell membrane protects the cell from outside forces. It consists of the lipid bilayer with embedded proteins

8. A
The Strong Nuclear Force is an attractive force that binds protons and neutrons and maintains the structure of the nucleus, and the Weak Nuclear Force is responsible for the radioactive beta decay and other subatomic reactions.

Note: The Weak Nuclear Force is so named because it is only effective for short distances. Nevertheless, it is through the Weak Nuclear Force that the sun provides us with energy by allowing one element to change into another element.[23]

9. D
Qualitative research deals with the quality, type or components of a group, substance, or mixture.

10. A
Adaptation is a trait that has evolved by natural selection.

11. A
A pH indicator measures hydrogen ions in a solution and show pH on a color scale.

12. B
The sun is the earth's primary source of energy.

13. B
The goal of quantitative research is to determine the relationship between one thing (an independent variable) and another (a dependent or outcome variable) in

a population.

14. C
A base is any substance that can accept a hydrogen ion and can react with fats to form soaps.

15. D
The dominant gene controls the expression of a trait.

16. B
Plants and animals are kingdoms. There are six recognized kingdoms: Animalia, Plantae, Protista, Fungi, Bacteria, and Archaea.

17. C
Organisms grouped into the Protista Kingdom include all unicellular organisms lacking a definite cellular arrangement such as bacteria and algae.

18. C
Indigestion is a common digestive affliction that most people suffer at one time or other.

19. D
Life functions are the biochemical and biophysical activities that all living systems must be able to carry out to maintain life.

20. C
Angina is frequently mistaken for a heart attack. Angina pectoris, commonly known as angina, is severe chest pain due to ischemia (a lack of blood, thus a lack of oxygen supply) of the heart muscle, generally due to obstruction or spasm of the coronary arteries (the heart's blood vessels). [24]

21. A
A biological class is a collection of similar or like living entities. Class has the same meaning in biology as rank. Common classes or ranks include species, order, and phylum.

22. A
Fats stay in the stomach the longest.

23. D
The periodic table as it is today, contains 118 elements.

24. D
A Punnett square resembles a game of tic-tac-toe, in which the genotypes of the

parents gametes are entered first, so that subsequent combinations can be calculated.

25. D
All of these statements are true.

    a. Prokaryotic cells include such organisms as E. coli and Streptococcus.

    b. Prokaryotic cells lack internal membranes and organelles.

    c. Prokaryotic cells break down food using cellular respiration and fermentation.

26. B
The process of converting observed phenomena into data is called Measurement.

27. A
The mass number of an atom is the total number of particles (protons and neutrons) that make it up.

28. B
Sublimation is the direct phase transition from solid to gas.

29. A
Exhalation is often accomplished by the abdominal muscles.

30. D
In Eukaryotic cells, the cell cycle is the cycle of events involving cell division, including mitosis, cytokinesis, and interphase.

31. D
All of the choices are correct.

    a. The genetic makeup, as distinguished from the physical appearance, of an organism or a group of organisms.

    b. The combination of alleles located on homologous chromosomes that determines a specific characteristic or trait.

    c. Is the inheritable information carried by all living organisms.

32. D
The blood is the primarily oxygenated through the work of the respiratory system.

33. B
Ribonucleic acid (RNA) is a chain of nucleotides that plays an important role in

the creation of new proteins.

34. A
A practical test designed with the intention that its results will be relevant to a particular theory or set of theories is an experiment.

35. C
Covalent or ionic bonds are considered "strong bonds."

36. A
The process by which the immune system adapts over time to be more efficient in recognizing pathogens is known as acquired immunity.

37. D
An organ is a group of tissues that perform a specific function or group of functions.

38. D
Reliability refers to the measure of an experiment's ability to yield the same or compatible results in different clinical experiments or statistical trials.

39. C
Each chemical element has a unique atomic number representing the number of protons in its nucleus.

40. C
The immune system is the system that protects the body from disease and infection.

41. D
The plasma membrane surrounds the cell and functions as an interface between the living interior of the cell and the nonliving exterior. [15]

42. C
An organelle is a specialized subunit of a cell with a specific function.

43. A
A solution with a pH value of less than 7 is acid. A pH value of 7 is neutral.

44. B
A catalyst is never changed in a chemical reaction.

45. A

The prediction that an observed difference is due to chance alone and not due to a systematic cause; this hypothesis is tested by statistical analysis, and accepted or rejected is the null hypothesis.

46. C

In science and engineering, the Accuracy of a measurement system is the degree of closeness of measurements of a quantity to its actual (true) value.

47. B

High blood pressure is a more common name for the circulatory system disease known as hypertension. Hypertension (HTN) or high blood pressure is a cardiac chronic medical condition in which the systemic arterial blood pressure is elevated.

48. B

The range of a distribution is the difference between the maximum value and the minimum value.

49. A

Statistical correlation is a statistical technique which determines if two variables are related.

50. A

In statistical analysis, the mean is the mathematical average of a set of numbers.

51. A

An Atom is the basic or fundamental particle of any matter or element.

52. C

When acid and base react, they neutralize each other properties to form salt and water.

53. B

The horizontal rows from right to left of the periodic table are known as periods and elements on a row share the same number of electron shells.

54. D

Oxidation and reduction reactions are each just half of a redox reaction and both occur simultaneously, because the exact electrons lost in oxidation is what is gained in reduction.

55. B
The elements on the periodic table can be classified as metals, metalloids and non-metals. Most of the elements on the table can be classified as metals.

56. D
All acids contain hydrogen. When acids react with most metals, the metals displace the hydrogen and hydrogen is produced.

57. B
Vertical columns on the periodic table are called groups. There are 18 groups on the table. Elements on the same group each have the same number of electrons on their outermost shell.

58. C
Redox is a complete reaction comprising oxidation and reduction reactions that are each only half of the complete reaction. The same exact electrons lost in oxidation are what are gained in reduction.

59. A
A chemical compound is a chemical substance comprising atoms from two or more elements in a specific ration as expressed in the chemical formula i.e., H2O

60. B
Acids turns blue litmus paper to red, base turns red litmus paper to blue.

Conclusion

CONGRATULATIONS! You have made it this far because you have applied yourself diligently to practicing for the exam and no doubt improved your potential score considerably! Getting into a good school is a huge step in a journey that might be challenging at times but will be many times more rewarding and fulfilling. That is why being prepared is so important.

Study then Practice and then Succeed!

Good Luck!

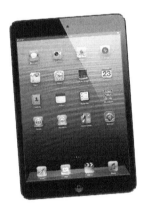

FREE Ebook Version

Download a FREE Ebook version of the publication!

Suitable for tablets, iPad, iPhone, or any smart phone.

**Go to
http://tinyurl.com/peuabux**

Register for Free Updates and More Practice Test Questions

Register your purchase at

www.test-preparation.ca/register.html for fast and convenient access to updates, errata, free test tips and more practice test questions.

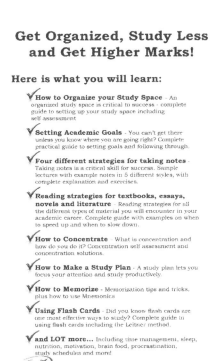
Get Organized, Study Less and Get Higher Marks!

Here is what you will learn:

- How to Organize your Study Space

- Four different strategies for taking notes

- Reading strategies for textbooks, essays, novels and literature

- How to Concentrate - What is concentration and how do you do it!

- Using Flash Cards - Complete guide to using flash cards including the Leitner method.

and LOT more... Including time management, sleep, nutrition, motivation, brain food, procrastination, study schedules and more!

Go to https://www.createspace.com/4060298

Enter Code LYFZGQB5 for 25% off!

NOTES

Text where noted below is used under the Creative Commons Attribution-ShareAlike 3.0 License

http://en.wikipedia.org/wiki/Wikipedia:Text_of_Creative_Commons_Attribution-ShareAlike_3.0_Unported_License

[1] Immune System. In *Wikipedia*. Retrieved November 12, 2010 from, en.wikipedia.org/wiki/Immune_system.

[2] White Blood Cell. In Wikipedia. Retrieved November 12, 2010 from en.wikipedia.org/wiki/White_blood_cell.

[3] Convection. In *Wikipedia*. Retrieved November 12, 2010 from en.wikipedia.org/wiki/Convection.

[4] Herr, N. (2008). The Sourcebook for Teaching Science: Strategies, Activities, and Instructional Resources. San Francisco, CA: John Wiley & Sons, Inc.

[5] Tight Junction. In *Wikipedia*. Retrieved November 12, 2010 from http://en.wikipedia.org/wiki/Tight_junction.

[6] Mechanical Energy (n.d.) Britannica Encyclopedia Online. Retrieved from www.britannica.com/EBchecked/topic/.../mechanical-energy.

[7] Biology. In Wikipedia. Retrieved May 10, 2012 from http://en.wikipedia.org/wiki/Biology.

[8] Chemistry. In Wikipedia. Retrieved May 10, 2012 from http://en.wikipedia.org/wiki/Chemistry.

[9] Infectious Disease. In *Wikipedia*. Retrieved November 12, 2010 from en.wikipedia.org/wiki/Infectious_disease.

[10] Virus. In *Wikipedia*. Retrieved November 12, 2010 from en.wikipedia.org/wiki/Virus.

[11] Thunderstorm. In *Wikipedia*. Retrieved November 12, 2010 from en.wikipedia.org/wiki/Thunderstorm.

[12] Meteorology. In *Wikipedia*. Retrieved November 12, 2010 from en.wikipedia.org/wiki/Outline_of_meteorology.

[13] U.S. Navy Seal. In *Wikipedia*. Retrieved November 12, 2010 from en.wikipedia.org/wiki/United_States_Navy_SEALs.

[14] What Causes DNA Mutations? (n.d.) Learn.Genetics http://learn.genetics.utah.edu/archive/sloozeworm/mutationbg.html

[15] Cell Membrane. In *Wikipedia*. Retrieved November 12, 2010 from http://en.wikipedia.org/wiki/Cell_membrane.

[16] Thoracic Diaphram. In Wikipedia. Retrieved January 2, 2012 from http://en.wikipedia.org/wiki/Thoracic_diaphragm.

[17] Brimblecombe, S., Gallannaugh, D., & Thompson, C. (1998). QPB Science Encyclopedia: An A to Z Guide to Everything You Need to Know About Science. New York, NY: Helicon Publishing Group Ltd.

[18] Arrythmia. In Wikipedia. Retrieved January 2, 2012 from http://en.wikipedia.org/wiki/Arrythmia

[19] Emphysema. In Wikipedia. Retrieved Jan 2, 2012 from http://en.wikipedia.org/wiki/Emphysema.

[20] Respiratory System. In *Wikipedia*. Retrieved November 12, 2010 from en.wikipedia. org/wiki/Respiratory_system.

[21] Mythology. In *Wikipedia*. Retrieved November 12, 2010 from en.wikipedia.org/wiki/ Mythology.

[22] Circulatory System. In *Wikipedia*. Retrieved November 12, 2010 from en.wikipedia. org/wiki/Circulatory_system

[23] The Four Fundamental Forces. (n.d.) Oracle Education Foundation. Retrieved from http:// library.thinkquest.org/27930/forces.htm

[24] Angina. In Wikipedia. Retrieved January 20, 2013 from http://en.wikipedia.org/wiki/Angina.

Made in the USA
Lexington, KY
13 May 2018